Knee Arthroplasty Handbook

Knee Arthroplasty Handbook

Techniques in Total Knee and Revision Arthroplasty

Editors

Giles R. Scuderi, M.D.
Insall Scott Kelly Institute New York, New York

Alfred J. Tria, Jr., M.D.
Orthopaedic Center of New Jersey Somerset, New Jersey

With 75 Figures

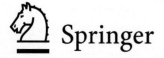 Springer

Giles R. Scuderi, M.D.
Insall Scott Kelly Institute
178 East 85th Street
New York, NY 10028

Alfred J. Tria, Jr., M.D.
Orthopaedic Center of New Jersey
1527 State Highway 27, Suite 1300
Somerset, NJ 08873 USA

Cover illustration: See Figure 7.7.

Library of Congress Control Number: 2005938493

ISBN-10: 0-387-30730-3
ISBN-13: 978-0387-307305

Printed on acid-free paper.

Printed in the United States of America.   (BS/MVY)

9 8 7 6 5 4 3 2 1

springer.com

◆

This book is dedicated to
our mentor,
John N. Insall, M.D.

◆

Preface

Knee Arthroplasty Handbook: Techniques in Total Knee and Revision Arthroplasty has been developed as a quick reference book for surgeons performing total knee replacement. Following completion of our previous book, *Surgical Techniques in Total Knee Arthroplasty*, we looked back retrospectively and condensed the material. We selected chapters that have a direct bearing on the surgical technique, such as instrumentation, correction of deformity, implant selection, revision arthroplasty and management of complications. We feel that these selected chapters, left in their original format, are an excellent summary of the topics at hand. The techniques are completely up to date and the manual approach should make it easier to obtain specific information in a minimal amount of time. This text should be a valuable assistance to medical students and residents who are attempting to develop an early expertise in total knee arthroplasty.

Giles R. Scuderi, MD
Alfred J. Tria, MD
November 2005

Contents

Preface vii
Contributors xi

1   The Basic Principles 1
GILES R. SCUDERI

2   Instrumentation in Total Knee Arthroplasty 7
ALFRED J. TRIA, JR.

3   Medial Release for Fixed-Varus Deformity 25
DAVID J. YASGUR, GILES R. SCUDERI, and
JOHN N. INSALL

4   Lateral Release for Fixed-Valgus Deformity 41
FRANKIE M. GRIFFIN, GILES R. SCUDERI, and
JOHN N. INSALL

5   Flexion Contracture in Total Knee Arthroplasty 57
PAUL A. LOTKE and R.G. SIMON

6   Cement in Primary Total Knee Arthroplasty 70
ALFRED J. TRIA, JR.

7   Cementless Total Knee Arthroplasty 80
AARON A. HOFMANN and DAVID F. SCOTT

8   Three-Step Technique for Revision Total Knee
Arthroplasty 104
KELLY G. VINCE and DANIEL A. OAKES

9   Classification of Bone Defects: Femur and Tibia 116
GERARD A. ENGH

10   Constrained Total Knee Designs for Revision
Arthroplasty 133
JAMES RAND and WILLIAM MARTIN

11   Two-Stage Reimplantation for Infection 150
GILES R. SCUDERI and HENRY D. CLARKE

12 Acute and Chronic Rupture of the Quadriceps Tendon
Treated with Direct Repair   154
ROBERT E. BOOTH and FRANK P. FEMINO

13 Management of the Patella Tendon Disruptions in
Total Knee Arthroplasty   158
GILES R. SCUDERI and BRIAN C. DE MUTH

14 Revision of Periprosthetic Femur Fractures   169
ROBERT E. BOOTH and DAVID G. NAZARIAN

15 Revision Arthroplasty for Tibial Periprosthetic
Fractures   175
WAYNE G. PAPROSKY, TODD D. SEKUNDIAK, and
JOHN KRONICK

Index   191

Contributors

ROBERT E. BOOTH, JR., M.D.
Chief of Orthopaedics
Pennsylvania Hospital
Philadelphia, PA, USA

HENRY D. CLARKE, M.D.
Attending Orthopaedic Surgeon
The Mayo Clinic
Scottsdale, AZ, USA

BRIAN C. DEMUTH, M.D.
The Insall Scott Kelly Institute
Beth Israel Medical Center
New York, NY, USA

GERARD A. ENGH, M.D.
Associate Clinical Professor
University of Maryland Medical School
Baltimore, MD, USA
President
Anderson Orthopedic Institute
Alexandria, VA, USA

FRANK P. FEMINO, M.D.
Department of Orthopaedics
Pennsylvania Hospital
Philadelphia, PA, USA

FRANKIE M. GRIFFIN, M.D.
The Insall Scott Kelly Institute
Orthopedic Surgeon
Van Buran, ARK, USA

AARON A. HOFMANN, M.D.
Professor, Department of Orthopaedics
University of Utah
Salt Lake City, UT, USA

JOHN N. INSALL, M.D. (1930–2000)
Clinical Professor of Orthopaedic Surgery
Albert Einstein College of Medicine
Bronx, NY, USA
Director and Founder
The Insall Scott Kelly Institute
New York, NY, USA

JOHN KRONICK, M.D.
Central DuPage Hospital
Winfield, IL, USA

PAUL A. LOTKE, M.D.
Professor, Department of Orthopaedics
University of Pennsylvania Hospital
Philadelphia, PA, USA

WILLIAM MARTIN, M.D.
Department of Orthopaedic Surgery
Mayo Clinic
Scottsdale, AZ, USA

DAVID G. NAZARIAN, M.D.
Department of Orthopaedic Surgery
Pennsylvania Hospital
Philadelphia, PA, USA

DANIEL A. OAKES, M.D.
Department of Orthopaedics
University of Louisville
Louisville, KY, USA

WAYNE G. PAPROSKY, M.D.
Department of Adult Joint Reconstruction
Rusk-Presbyterian-St. Lukes Medical Center
Chicago, IL, USA

JAMES ALAN RAND, M.D.
Department of Orthopaedic Surgery
Mayo Clinic
Scottsdale, AZ, USA

DAVID F. SCOTT, M.D.
Department of Orthopaedics
University of Utah
Salt Lake City, UT, USA

GILES R. SCUDERI, M.D.
Attending Orthopedic Surgeon
Lenox Hill Hospital
New York, NY, USA
Director, The Insall Scott Kelly Institute
New York, NY, USA
Assistant Clinical Professor of Orthopaedic Surgery
Albert Einstein College of Medicine
Bronx, NY, USA

TODD D. SEKUNDIAK M.D.
Section of Orthopaedics
University of Manitoba
Winnipeg, Manitoba, Canada

R.G. SIMON, M.D.
Department of Orthopaedics
University of Pennsylvania Hospital
Philadelphia, PA, USA

ALFRED J. TRIA, M.D.
Clinical Professor of Orthopaedic Surgery
Robert Wood Johnson Medical School
Orthopaedic Center of New Jersey
Somerset, NJ, USA

KELLY G. VINCE, M.D.
Associate Professor
Department of Orthopaedics
University of Louisville
Louisville, KY, USA

DAVID J. YASGUR, M.D.
Katonah Medical Group
Katonah, NY, USA

Chapter 1
The Basic Principles

Giles R. Scuderi

In primary total knee arthroplasty, whether a posterior cruciate-retaining or posterior cruciate-substituting design is implanted, the clinical results are influenced by the surgical technique. Adherence to the basic principles of the surgical technique ensures a successful outcome.

The goal of primary total knee arthroplasty is to reestablish the normal mechanical axis with a stable prosthesis that is well fixed (Fig. 1.1). This is achieved by both the bone resection and the soft tissue balance. The femoral component should be aligned with 5 to 10 degrees valgus angulation in the coronal plane and 0 to 10 degrees of flexion in the sagittal plane. The tibia should be resected at 90 ± 2 degrees to the long axis of the tibia in the coronal plane. In the sagittal plane, the posterior slope is dictated by the prosthetic design, but it appears preferable to recreate the posterior slope of the natural tibia.

Regardless of prosthetic design there are three basic bone cuts in primary total knee arthroplasty: the proximal tibia, the distal femur, and the posterior femur (Fig. 1.2). Each one influences the arthroplasty in a different manner (Table 1.1). Usually the amount of bone resected corresponds to the thickness of the component being implanted. Resection of the proximal tibia influences both the flexion and extension gaps and is replaced by the tibial component. The more tibial bone resected, the thicker the tibial component. Resection of the distal femur selectively influences the extension gap. Usually the distal femur is resected 9 to 10 mm from the unaffected or normal side, which in the case of a varus knee is the lateral femoral condyle. This concept of removing as much bone as being replaced by the femoral component helps to reassure reestablishment of the joint line. Over-resection of the distal femur creates an extension gap that is larger than the flexion gap resulting in recurvatum, whereas under-resection creates a flexion contracture. Resection of the posterior femur selectively influences the flexion space. If the flexion gap is larger than the extension gap,

$$\text{Alignment} \quad \leftarrow \quad \underset{\downarrow}{\overset{\uparrow}{\text{Total Knee Arthroplasty}}} \quad \rightarrow \quad \text{Stability}$$

Fixation

Kinematics

FIGURE 1.1. The goals of total knee arthroplasty.

then posterior flexion instability will occur. It is recommended that the amount of bone resected be replaced by the implant.

There is a fourth cut that seems to receive less attention. The anterior femoral resection influences both the flexion space and the patellofemoral joint. The amount of bone resected from the ante-

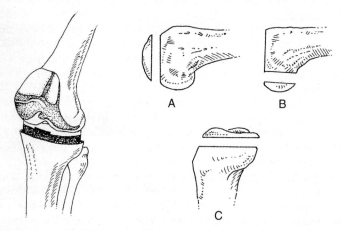

A   B

C

FIGURE 1.2. The three basic cuts in total knee arthroplasty include the distal femur (A), the posterior femur (B), and the proximal tibia (C). Correct positioning and spacing of these cuts will ensure a stable and well-aligned prosthesis.

TABLE 1.1. The basic principles of total knee arthroplasty

1. Restoration of the mechanical axis
2. Restoration of the joint line
3. Balance of the soft tissues
4. Equalize flexion and extension gaps
5. Restore patellofemoral alignment and mechanics

rior femur is dependent upon sizing of the femur and position of the anteroposterior cutting guide. Under-resection of the anterior femur is caused by an inappropriately large femoral component or by anterior placement of the correct size component with excessive posterior resection. This leads to overstuffing of the patellofemoral joint, which may possibly lead to limited motion and patellofemoral dysfunction. Conversely, over-resection of the anterior condyles may result in notching of the distal femur.

The ligament releases, to correct fixed angular deformities, are discussed elsewhere in this text and should be reviewed, but the basic principles will be highlighted. For the fixed-varus deformity, the medial soft tissue release includes the deep medial collateral ligament, the posteriomedial corner (including the semitendinosus), and the superficial medial collateral ligament. Correction of a fixed-valgus deformity tends to be sequential with release of the posterolateral capsule, the iliotibial band, and the lateral collateral ligament. If possible, it is preferable to preserve the integrity of the popliteus tendon in order to maintain flexion stability. Whatever the fixed deformity, balancing of the tight contracted soft tissues is critical in reestablishing the normal mechanical axis of the knee.

Of prime importance is establishing equal flexion and extension gaps (Fig. 1.3). Anteroposterior stability depends on balanced flexion and extension gaps. These gaps are influenced by femoral component sizing, asymmetry of the flexion space, flexion contracture, and release of the posterior cruciate ligament. Each variable affects the knee in a different way. Failure to address these issues may result in posterior subluxation or dislocation, irrespective of prosthetic design. It is a misconception that proper soft tissue releases that restore the mechanical axis to neutral in extension will ensure stability in flexion. As each variable is reviewed, their influence will be better understood.

Matching the femoral component to the anteroposterior dimension of the femur has always been recommended. When the femur measures in-between sizes, it may be preferable to downsize the femoral component. In this situation, an anterior-referencing system will resect more bone from the posterior femur enlarging the flexion gap, whereas a posterior-referencing system will resect more bone from the anterior femur resulting in an anterior notch (Fig. 1.4). The ideal system should allow the additional bone resection to be divided between the anterior and posterior condyles. Slight flexion of the distal femoral resection avoids anterior notching and permits blending of the anterior femur. There may be situations in which upsizing of the femoral component is preferable,

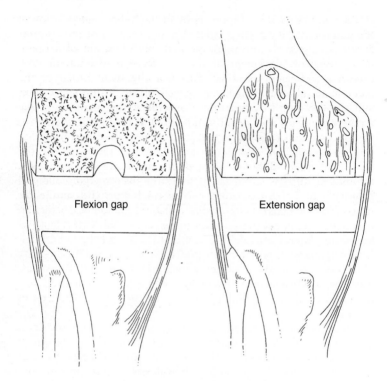

Flexion gap   Extension gap

FIGURE 1.3. The flexion gap must equal the extension gap.

this is usually the case with a wide distal femur whose anteroposterior measurement is within 1 to 2 mm of the next larger femoral component.

External rotation of the femoral component has always been advocated. Whether the rotation is set at a predetermined 3 degrees, referenced off the posterior condyles or set in line with the epicondylar axis, a certain amount of external rotation is desirable. The femoral epicondylar axis is a reliable and reproducible landmark for setting femoral component rotation. Following soft tissue balancing, setting the femoral component along the epicondylar axis creates a balanced rectangular space. In addition to its influence on patellar tracking, internal rotation of the femoral component must be avoided because this will cause asymmetry of the flexion space. This asymmetry results in a trapezoidal flexion space that would be tight on the medial side and loose on the lateral side.

Asymmetry of the flexion space can also be related to over-release of a valgus deformity. As discussed elsewhere in this text, there are several techniques described for correction of a fixed-valgus deformity. Although complete release of the lateral supporting structures will correct the axial alignment in extension, over-release will result in an asymmetry of the flexion space. The resultant trapezoidal space would be larger on the lateral side than on the medial side. Correction of the valgus deformity should be sequential, lengthening the lateral soft tissues and attempting to maintain flexion stability.

Following standard resection of the femur and tibia, a knee with a preoperative flexion contracture will probably have a flexion-extension space imbalance. The flexion space would be larger than the extension space. Although it might be appealing to use a thinner tibial polyethylene component, this would cause

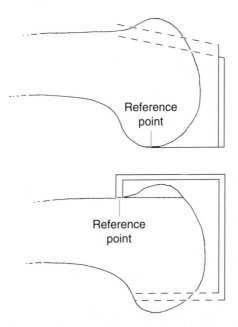

FIGURE 1.4. When sizing the femur the level of resection can be referenced from the posterior or anterior femur. The posterior reference point causes variation in the anterior resection when the femur measures in between sizes, while an anterior reference point causes variation in the posterior cuts.

flexion instability. The correct management of this situation should be a posterior capsule release and resection of additional bone from the distal femur so that the extension space equals the flexion space.

Finally, correct preparation of the patella ensures improved performance of the extensor mechanism and reduces the incidence of complications. The preparation of the patella includes a measured resection that is parallel to the anterior cortex. The bone-patellar component composite should be as thick as the original patella. Even though lateralization of the femoral and tibial components are advocated, the patellar component should be medialized. The assessment of patella tracking is judged by the rule of "no thumbs." Further details of patellar preparation will be discussed in later chapters.

Adhering to these basic principles in both the simple and complex cases ensures a successful outcome.

Chapter 2
Instrumentation in Total Knee Arthroplasty

Alfred J. Tria, Jr.

INTRODUCTION

In the early 1970s the total condylar knee arthroplasty was designed at the Hospital for Special Surgery and emphasized the concepts of ligament balance and knee alignment.[1] After the introduction of polymethylmethacrylate, there was a rapid increase in design work because the major obstacle of fixation was relieved. Although the knee implant designs continued to undergo refinement, instrumentation lagged significantly behind the design technology. This dichotomy occurred because the emphasis was given to the development of better anatomic and biomechanical prostheses that could take advantage of the new fixation and improve upon the early loosening and increase the range of motion. The technique for the implantation of the knee was not a central issue. Thus, instruments were designed after the prostheses had been developed and oftentimes were not even available for the initial surgical procedures.

In the 1980s the knee designs became more sophisticated and the concept of a cementless prosthesis was introduced.[2] The cementless components required more accurate bone cuts in order to increase the surface area of contact between the prosthesis and the bone. This placed a much greater demand upon the instrumentation and required a parallel technology to complete the prosthesis and the instruments as one unified system. It became evident that the results of the new implants were dependent both upon the design rationale of the prosthesis and the surgical technique. It was no longer acceptable to rely upon the "surgeon's eye" to establish proper positioning of the implant. Implant design and instrument design became equally important.

PRINCIPALS OF INSTRUMENTATION

Tibiofemoral Alignment

The overall alignment of the knee must be in 5 to 10 degrees of anatomic valgus. The alignment is determined by the position of both the femoral and tibial components in the coronal plane of the joint. There are two basic schools of thought concerning the position of the knee joint.[3,4] The most popular school references the *mechanical axis* of the lower leg. The tibial cut is made perpendicular to the tibial shaft and the femoral cut is made parallel to the mechanical axis of the femur (i.e., the line drawn from the femoral head through the middle of the tibia and through the middle of the ankle). The *anatomic alignment* references the mechanical axis of the lower leg but allows for the fact that the proximal tibial plateau is actually in a few degrees of varus. In this system the tibial cut is set anatomically (i.e., in 2 to 3 degrees of varus) and the femoral cut is made parallel to the mechanical axis with the addition of the 2 or 3 degrees. Hungerford and Krackow popularized this concept hoping to improve knee arthroplasty with greater anatomic precision (Fig. 2.1).

The Femoral Component
The preceding discussion has only considered the angular relationship of the femur and the tibia in the coronal plane. The instruments must align *each component* in the sagittal, coronal, and horizontal planes. The femoral component should include a valgus angle of 4 to 6 degrees, should be centered on the end of the femoral shaft with respect to the anteroposterior plane, should not be significantly flexed or extended, and should include external rotation of 3 to 4 degrees.

The femoral valgus angle can be referenced with respect to the femoral shaft. The anterior to posterior position and the external rotation can be verified with respect to the posterior condylar axis, the anterior cortex of the shaft of the femur, the intramedullary canal, the epicondyles, and the flexion gap. Each of the references has an individual variability. The posterior femoral condyles are easily defined. However, as the varus or valgus deformity of the knee increases the posterior aspect of the medial condyle (in varus) and the lateral condyle (in valgus) can become deficient. With this atrophy, the anterior to posterior thickness will be underestimated and the femoral cuts will be internally rotated in the valgus deformity and externally rotated in the varus deformity if the posterior condylar axis is the primary reference (Fig. 2.2). The anterior cortex of the femur is readily available for referencing.[5] Because the lateral femoral condyle rises higher than the medial condyle in the femoral sulcus area, the surgeon must choose between the high lateral referencing or the low medial referencing. If the anterior cut is elevated, the forces in the patellofemoral joint will be increased because of the increased distance of the patella from the center of

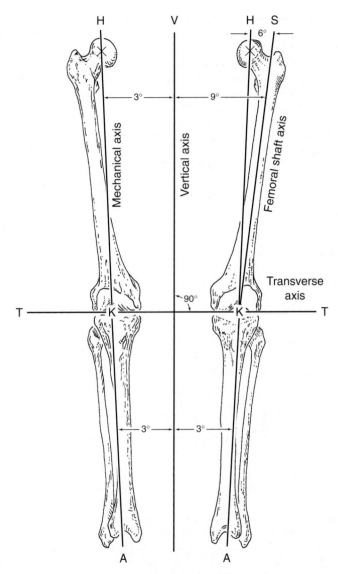

FIGURE 2.1. The figure on the left illustrates the mechanical axis of the knee. The figure on the right shows the femoral anatomic axis with the tibial reference line drawn to allow for the anatomic varus of the tibia of 3 degrees.

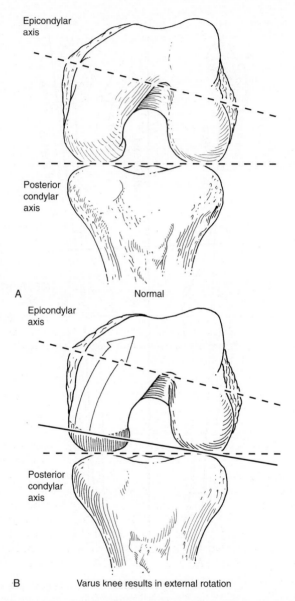

FIGURE 2.2. (A) The relationship of the posterior condylar axis and the epicondylar axis. (B) The varus knee presents with an atrophic medial femoral condyle, especially posteriorly. This can result in increased external rotation of the femoral component if the posterior condylar axis is used as the only reference point.

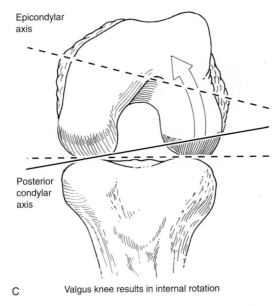

Valgus knee results in internal rotation

C

FIGURE 2.2. *Continued.* (C) The valgus knee presents with an atrophic lateral femoral condyle, especially posteriorly. This can result in increased internal rotation of the femoral component if the posterior condylar axis is used as the only reference point.

rotation of the knee. Anterior positioning of the femoral component will also increase the flexion space. If the cut is lowered on the anterior surface, there is the chance of femoral notching. A notch defect of 1 or 2 mm is probably not significant; however, deeper defects can be associated with supracondylar fracture. If all femoral cuts are referenced from the anterior cortex despite the size of the chosen component, the smaller component will increase the flexion gap, perhaps out of proportion to the extension gap, and may remove an undesirable amount of bone. The larger femoral component will decrease the flexion gap without a proportionate effect on the extension space (Fig. 2.3).

The intramedullary canal of the femur is a stable referencing point, especially in the revision case in which there can be significant bone deficits and loss of palpable bone landmarks. The canal helps with the anteroposterior position and with the valgus distal

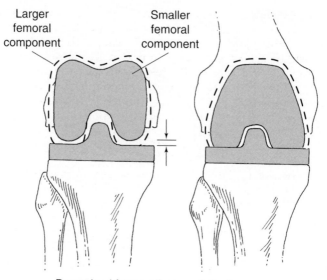

Downsized femur affects *only* flexion gap

FIGURE 2.3. The flexion gap is affected by the size of the femoral component without significant effects on the extension space.

cut. The intramedullary referencing rod is most accurate if the length is increased to engage the isthmus of the femoral shaft. The accuracy can also be increased if the width of the intramedullary rod is increased to engage both the medial and lateral cortex of the femur. The intramedullary canal itself does not provide good rotational referencing.

The epicondyles are especially helpful with respect to rotational positioning; however, it is sometimes difficult to identify the exact center point, most especially of the medial epicondyle.[6,7] Rubash has reported some excellent anatomic studies comparing the epicondylar axis with the posterior condylar axis and he has shown that they do indeed correlate with each other.[8] The transepicondylar axis of the distal femur does represent a reproducible landmark. The epicondyles are identified and the component is rotated until it is parallel to the axis. This reference is based solely upon the femoral anatomy, much the same as the posterior condyles. The surgeon should not confuse the rotational positioning of the femoral component with the flexion-extension gap in reference to the tibial component. With this technique the balancing is considered as a completely separate issue. The flexion gap technique for femoral rotation is based upon the reference to the tibial cut with the *collateral ligaments balanced* in flexion. The knee is distracted in flexion after the tibial cut has been completed. The collateral ligaments are balanced equally and the posterior femoral cut is made parallel to the proximal tibial cut surface to create a rectangular space (the "gap" technique as described by Insall) (Fig. 2.4).[9] This technique assures ligament balance in flexion but if either collateral is abnormally tight or lax, the femoral rotation can be incorrect and interfere with patellar tracking.

The rotational alignment of the femoral component effects both the tracking of the patella and the balance of the collateral ligaments in flexion. The sulcus of the femoral component must articulate with the patella and maintain normal contact from extension to full flexion. Internal rotation of the femoral component will allow the patella to track laterally with respect to the femoral sulcus. Internal rotation will also tighten the medial flexion space

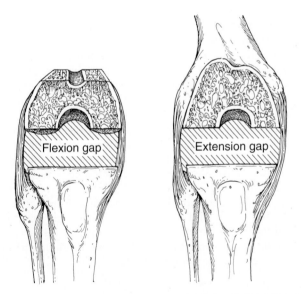

FIGURE 2.4. With the collateral ligaments balanced in flexion, the posterior femoral cut can be made parallel to the proximal tibia to create a rectangular space in flexion which must then be matched in extension.

and open up the lateral flexion space gap. External rotation of the femoral component favors the tracking of the patella; however, if the external rotation is excessive, the patella can track medially and the flexion gap can become too large on the medial side and too small on the lateral.

The Tibial Component
The tibial component must also be considered as a separate entity similar to the femoral component. Most tibial cuts are perpendicular to the tibial shaft in the coronal plane unless the knee system incorporates an anatomic 3 or 4 degrees of varus. In the sagittal plane the tibial cut is usually perpendicular or includes a slight posterior angulation to help with the flexion range of motion improving the rollback of the femoral component on the tibial surface. Many knee systems include a slight posterior angulation in the polyethylene surface and cut the tibial plateau at a 90-degree angle. If the slope is built into the polyethylene, there must be some thinning of the polyethylene from the anterior to the posterior aspect of the surface. With the thinner inserts, it is possible to approach the critical thickness of 6 mm or less. Thus, some designs incorporate the slope in the tibial cut and then implant a polyethylene that is of uniform thickness from anterior to posterior and avoid the issue of changing polyethylene thickness.

The tibia must also be rotated in the horizontal plane with respect to the tibial tubercle.[6,7] The tibial rotation is slightly less complicated than the femoral (Fig. 2.4). The tibial tubercle is the major landmark for referencing. Most component systems center upon the tubercle unless there is a marked external or, less commonly, internal rotation of the tibial tuberosity. With abnormal tubercle anatomy, the tibial rotation is usually determined with respect to the femoral component in the flexed position and then referenced in extension to check the entire range of motion. It can become difficult to choose the proper position when the existing tubercle is markedly rotated. If the tibial tray is internally rotated, the patella will track with the patellar ligament and tend to shift laterally. If the tray is externally rotated, the patella will track more centrally but the tibiofemoral contact will not be anatomic and the rotational torque can lead to loosening or wear.

The Patellar Component
As the technology for knee arthroplasty improves, the last area of difficulty is the patellofemoral articulation. The patella must track centrally throughout the range of motion despite the individual

position of the femoral and tibial components. Soft tissue procedures and/or tubercle osteotomies are sometimes required to
center the patella on the femoral sulcus.[10,11] The thickness of the
patella has become a point of concern and instruments can be
helpful with this problem. Although the literature is scant at the
present time, there is a tendency to favor decreasing the overall
thickness of the resurfaced patella versus the original presenting
thickness. Thinning the patella brings the component closer to the
center of rotation of the knee and decreases the forces on the
surface, hopefully decreasing wear and fracture. Most surgeons
favor retaining a minimum of 10 mm of the original patellar bed.
The patellar cut should be parallel to the anterior cortical surface
and the thickness should be equal to or less than the original thickness. The patella can also be placed eccentrically on the cut bed.
The author favors a central position; however, some groups recommend medial placement of the patella to favor better tracking
on the femoral surface.

If the patellar component is facetted, the alignment becomes
even more important. The patella may track centrally; yet, there
may still be an element of torque if the facets are rotated out of
position versus the femoral condyles. The problem of facet alignment can be somewhat corrected if the patella is a mobile-bearing
surface that can rotate throughout the range of motion. The
mobile-bearing designs require a metal baseplate and often will
increase the overall thickness of the patella leading to increased
forces and possible increased wear.

INSTRUMENTATION

Cutting Instruments

Early knee arthroplasty was performed with simple hand imple-
ments and without sophisticated cutting guides. With the introduction of power tools, the cuts became more reproducible and the
surgeons demanded better guides. Cutting blocks were introduced
and the sawblade rested upon the block for support and direction
(Fig. 2.5). Cutting slots were then introduced to grasp the blade
better and protect it from roaming across the guide block. The slots
took the sawblade to the best accuracy that it could afford. Then,
the concept of frames was introduced. The frame can be applied
to the bone and the cutting blade is locked into a slot for the various
cuts. The advantage of the frame is the single application with
several cuts completed at the same step (Fig. 2.6). Multiple blocks
and slots lead to multiple opportunities for the introduction of
inaccuracies. The frame eliminates several steps and, thus, elimi-

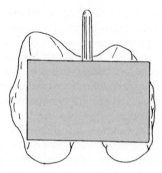

FIGURE 2.5. The femoral cutting block is pinned on the distal surface with proper rotation.

nates more of the chances for inaccurate cuts. The next logical step was to introduce rotary blades to be used with the frames. The rotary blade eliminates the wobble of the long oscillating blade, decreases the temperature of the cut bone surface, and controls the depth of the cut. At the present time the sawblade with the cutting

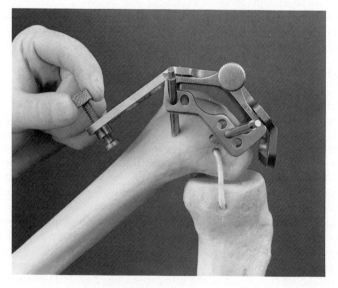

FIGURE 2.6. An external frame applied to the distal femur allows all of the subsequent cuts to be completed with a single reference point.

slots still represents the gold standard in knee arthroplasty. The author favors the use of the frames with rotary blades and looks to the future for greater improvement of these devices.

Although lasers have gained a great deal in other specialties, open knee procedures do not favor the user of the laser. The electrocautery remains the primary device for hemostasis and the power tools cut the bone quite accurately and acceptably.

There have been some attempts to apply robotic arms to the knee surgery and this may become more popular in the future when the instruments become more accurate and lock the cutting devices into place about the bone. It is also difficult for the arm to use the standard bone landmarks that are presently used. When the landmarks become more accurate and reproducible, it may be more appropriate to visit this technology again.

Instrument Design

The designer's choice of anatomic references concerning alignment and balance of the knee arthroplasty components significantly affects the type of instrument that is subsequently designed. The discussion earlier outlines the multitude of parameters that are available for referencing each component.

During the arthroplasty, the surgeon must address the femur, the tibia, and the patella as separate entities and then as an integrated unit. Various systems begin on the femoral or the tibial side. With either approach, the considerations are the same but are addressed at different points during the surgical procedure. This chapter will begin with the tibial preparation and proceed to the femur and then to the patella.

Tibial Preparation

The instruments for the tibial preparation are based upon intramedullary or extramedullary referencing. Because the anterior prominence of the tibial shaft and the malleoli of the ankle joint are usually readily palpable, extramedullary rods for the tibia are very reliable. The tibial tubercle and the fibular head are usually available for referencing except in the worst revision cases. The initial tibial cut is usually perpendicular to the shaft with a slight posterior angulation according to the system that is being used. The tibial jigs attach to the anterior tibia in line with the tubercle and include either a capture slot to enclose the oscillating sawblade or a cutting block upon which the sawblade rests. Capture slots control the oscillating sawblade but tend to block the full view of the underlying bone. Cutting blocks allow more complete visualization of the bone surface but they also allow more sawblade deviation. The tibial cutting slots can accommodate angled cuts to prepare the plateau surface to accept a wedge attached to the tibial tray. Rotary blade power cutters are presently being considered to fashion the tibia and femur. These devices create significant bone debris and require capture slots that often obscure the bone surface from the operating surgeon.

Intramedullary tibial jigs are also available for this primary cut. The tibial shaft is often too narrow for the rod, or the shaft is curved, or the proximal tibial surface requires offset from the central canal, making intramedullary placement difficult or sometimes impossible. Simmons studied the accuracy of the intramedullary devices and reported neutral alignment in 83% of the varus knees and only 37% of the valgus knees.[12] The major source of the difficulty was the tibial bowing, which was present in 66% of the valgus knees. He recommended preoperative long films or cross checking with external alignment in the genu valgus deformity (Table 2.1). The literature indicates that either the extramedullary or the intramedullary instruments are equally accurate for the tibial cut; however, the intramedullary technique may not be possible in the setting of the valgus knee.

Femoral Preparation

The femoral preparation is the more difficult portion of the knee arthroplasty. The femoral shaft is less visible and palpable than the tibia because of the bulk of the thigh musculature, the proximal arterial tourniquet, and the commonly associated thigh obesity. The femoral head is not a palpable landmark and the anterior superior iliac spine is often difficult to identify beneath the surgical drapes. The femoral shaft has the natural anterior bow and may also include a varus bow. Multiple studies have been performed to evaluate the accuracy of either the extramedullary or the

TABLE 2.1. The accuracy of the intramedullary and extramedullary tibial jigs varies in the reported literature

	Intramedullary	Extramedullary
Manning[17]	90%	—
Engh[15]	—	82%
Brys[18]	94%	85%
Dennis[20]	72%	88%
Laskin[21]	97%	—

TABLE 2.2. The published results of intramedullary and extramedullary femoral jigs clearly favor the intramedullary devices

	Intramedullary	Extramedullary
Manning[17]	90%	—
Engh[15]	87.5%	68.8%
Cates[19]	85.6%	72%
Siegel[22]	—	>2–3° (unacceptable)

intramedullary alignment rods (Table 2.2).[13–22] At the present time the intramedullary rod systems appear to be more helpful and can be checked with extramedullary backup. In 1988, Tillett and Engh compared extramedullary and intramedullary alignment systems for the distal femoral cut and found no significant difference.[13] The femoral head was located for the extramedullary system using a radio opaque marker with roentgenographic verification in the operating room before the procedure was undertaken. The authors admitted that the roentgenogram required greater time and that the intramedullary system was more expedient. The same authors subsequently published a comparative experience using similar techniques for both the extramedullary and intramedullary alignment guides.[15] They reported 87.5% correct alignment with the intramedullary system and only 68.8% correct with the extramedullary. They explained the difference in their two papers by indicating that in the newer paper they used longer X-ray cassettes for greater measuring accuracy. Second, they reported greater variation with larger discrepancies in the extramedullary group.

If the intramedullary canal of the femur is particularly large, it is possible to ream the canal eccentrically and insert the reference rod into the canal in an incorrect varus or valgus position. Bertin reviewed these possibilities and showed that a lengthened rod with an increased diameter helped to prevent some of the discrepancies (Fig. 2.7).[23] Once the intramedullary rod is properly placed, the distal end of the femur can be resected with the appropriate valgus angulation to reestablish the biomechanical axis of the lower extremity. The exact choice of the angle can be made with preoperative full-length standing films or with intraoperatively placed markers that are roentgenographically positioned and checked. Despite the modifications of the intramedullary devices, extramedullary confirmation of the component position is still advised during the operative procedure. The author does not rely upon full-length standing roentgenograms for the valgus align-

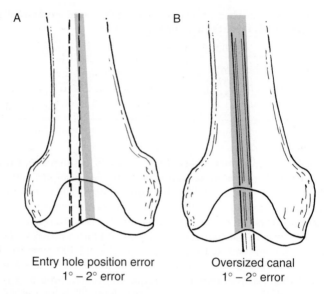

Entry hole position error
1° – 2° error

Oversized canal
1° – 2° error

FIGURE 2.7. The femoral hole on the left is eccentric and will lead to increased valgus. The intramedullary rod on the right is centrally placed but can shift into varus or valgus if the rod is too short.

ment. In the varus knee, the intramedullary guide is positioned and 4 degrees of valgus is set in place. In the valgus knee we chose 2 to 3 degrees of valgus for the intramedullary guide. With these choices we have found that the femorotibial angle is 5 to 10 degrees on the postoperative roentgenograms. This somewhat arbitrary angle assignment allows us to perform the arthroplasty in a timely fashion and to avoid significant malalignment.

Keying from the intramedullary rod helps to prevent flexion or extension of the femoral component. The intramedullary reference permits direct visualization of the anterior and posterior cortices and allows the surgeon to choose the anterior to posterior placement of the femoral component that is the best solution for the relationship of the patellofemoral joint and the tibiofemoral flexion gap.

Although the intramedullary femoral guide does appear to solve most of the femoral problems, the surgeon is still left with the choice of the rotational position. Except in the most deformed cases, the epicondyles of the femur are readily palpable. The difficulty with the epicondyles has been the problem of establishing the exact center of each prominence. Insall has contributed significant insight into the anatomy with his new epicondylar instruments and Rubash has shown that the medial epicondyle has a central depression that can be clearly identified if the overlying synovium is thoroughly removed.[8] The central depression can also be confirmed with a circle of marker dots that are placed about the base of the medial epicondylar prominence and then connected across to identify the center of the circle. Krackow's textbook refers to the epicondyles for the rotational alignment.[24] Whitesides' article identifies the anteroposterior axis of the femoral sulcus and relates this to the epicondyles and the posterior condylar axis (Fig. 2.1).[25] Rubash's work shows the relationship of the posterior condylar axis and the epicondylar axis and confirms the correlation between the two.[8]

Patellar Preparation

Instruments for cutting the patellar surface are still at the early design level. There are many surgeons who believe that the patella can be best cut with the power saw and a well-trained eye. Even though experience is one of the most valuable instruments, cutting guides can only help to improve the accuracy. The patella is most commonly cut with an oscillating saw locked into a capture slot or with the sawblade resting on a cutting block. It is true that the blade can wobble on the top of a block and can also angle in the cutting slot, if the slot is not made tight enough. There are also cutting devices that encircle the patella and then use a rotating type blade to remove the posterior surface. The holding devices are somewhat bulky and it is also true that the cutting device obscures the patella while the reaming is completed. At the present time, there is no ideal solution and resurfacing of the patella must be completed as accurately as possible. The author uses a rotating type blade and confirms the position in the middle of the reaming so that any necessary correction can be made before the entire procedure is completed with an off angle cut (Fig. 2.8).

Balancing the Knee

After the tibia and the femur have been appropriately prepared, the flexion and extension gaps must be equaled. At the present time, this soft tissue balancing is completed at full extension and at 90 degrees of flexion. Most knee systems do not incorporate an instrument to perform or confirm the balancing. Tensing devices have been introduced that spread the tibia and femur and allow measurements of the gaps that are established with the ligaments balanced. In the past, the instruments have been bulky and have not added precision beyond hand tensioning. Dr. Robert Booth has

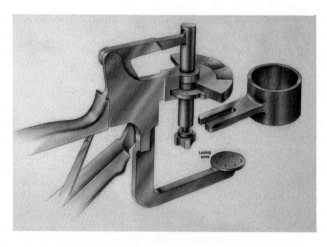

FIGURE 2.8. The patellar cutting guide.

developed a new tensor that establishes the soft tissue balance and predicts the size of the femoral component and the thickness of the tibial insert with a comparison from flexion to extension (Fig. 2.9). The author has had the opportunity to use the instrument with some early successes. If such a device can be refined, it may be possible to eliminate some of the guesswork that is involved in matching the flexion and extension spaces.

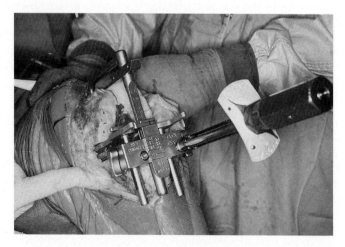

FIGURE 2.9. The tensor for flexion and extension balancing.

CONCLUSIONS

Instruments for total knee arthroplasty continue to be refined. Most systems develop the implants and the instruments at the same time with two different teams leading the investigations. There is no question that the more accurate the surgery performed, the better the result and longevity of the prosthesis.

At the present time, extramedullary tibial jigs, intramedullary femoral jigs, and patellar resurfacing with reference to the original thickness represent the standard. Instruments for the flexion and extension balancing are still in their infancy. The references and landmarks for the instruments will probably change over the next few years; however, the principle will remain the same.

References

1. Insall JN, Scott WN, Ranawat CS. The total condylar knee prosthesis: a report of two hundred and twenty cases. *J Bone Joint Surg*. 1979; 61(A):173–180.
2. Hungerford DS, Kenna RV. Preliminary experience with a porous coated total knee replacement used without cement. *Clin Orthop*. 1983; 176:95–107.
3. Moreland JR, Bassett LW, Hanker GJ. Radiographic analysis of the axial alignment of the lower extremity. *J Bone Joint Surg*. 1987; 69(A):745–749.
4. Krackow KA. *The Technique of Total Knee Arthroplasty*. St. Louis, Mo: The CV Mosby Company; 1990: Chap. 4, page 87.
5. Insall JN. *Surgery of the Knee*. 2nd ed. New York: Churchill Livingstone; 1993: Chap. 26, page 745.
6. Lotke PA, Ecker ML. Influence of positioning of prosthesis in total knee replacement. *J Bone Joint Surg*. 1977; 59(A):77–79.
7. Jiang C-C, Insall JN. Effect of rotation on the axial alignment of the femur. *Clin Orthop*. 1989; 248:50–56.
8. Berger RA, Rubash HE, Seel MJ, Thompson WH, Crossett LA. Determining the rotational alignment of the femoral component in total knee arthroplasty using the epicondylar axis. *Clin Orthop*. 1993; 286:40–47.
9. Insall JN. *Surgery of the Knee*. 2nd ed. New York: Churchill Livingstone; 1993: Chap. 26, page 746.
10. Wolff AM, Hungerford MD, Krackow KA, Jacobs MA. Osteotomy of the tibial tubercle during total knee replacement. *J Bone Joint Surg*. 1989; 6:848–856.
11. Whiteside LA, Ohl M. Tibial tubercle osteotomy for exposure of the difficult total knee arthroplasty. *Clin Orthop*. 1990; 260:6–9.
12. Simmons ED, Sullivan JA, Rackemann S, Scott RD. The accuracy of tibial intramedullary alignment devices in total knee arthroplasty. *J Arthroplasty*. 1991; 6:45–50.
13. Tillett ED, Engh GA, Petersen T. A comparative study of extramedullary and intramedullary alignment systems in total knee arthroplasty. *Clin Orthop*. 1988; 230:176–181.

14. Petersen TL, Engh GA. Radiographic assessment of knee alignment after total knee arthroplasty. *J Arthroplasty*. 1988; 3:67–72.

15. Engh GA, Petersen TL. Comparative experience with intramedullary and extramedullary alignment in total knee arthroplasty. *J Arthroplasty*. 1990; 5:1–8.

16. Whiteside LA, Summers RG. Anatomical landmarks for an intramedullary alignment system for total knee replacement. *Orthop Trans*. 1983; 7:546–547.

17. Manning M, Elloy M, Johnson R. The accuracy of intramedullary alignment in total knee replacement. *J Bone Joint Surg*. 1988; 70(B):852–858.

18. Brys DA, Lombardi AV, Mallory TH, Vaughn BK. A comparison of intramedullary and extramedullary alignment systems for tibial component placement in TKA. *Clin Orthop*. 1991; 263:175–179.

19. Cates HE, Ritter MA, Keating EM, Faris PM. Intramedullary versus extramedullary femoral alignment systems in total knee replacement. *Clin Orthop*. 1993; 286:32–39.

20. Dennis DA, Channer M, Susman MH, Stringer EA. Intramedullary versus extramedullary tibial alignment systems in total knee arthroplasty. *J Arthroplasty*. 1993; 8(1):43–47.

21. Laskin RS, Turtel A. The use of an intramedullary tibial alignment guide in TKR arthroplasty. *The American J of Knee Surgery*. 1989; 2(3):123–130.

22. Siegel JL, Shall LM. Femoral instrumentation using the anterosuperior iliac spine as a landmark in total knee arthroplasty. An anatomic study. *J Arthroplasty*. 1991; 6(4):317–320.

23. Bertin CB. Intramedullary instrumentation for total knee arthroplasty. In: Goldberg VM, ed. *Controversies in Total Knee Arthroplasty*. New York: Raven Press, Ltd., 1991; Chap. 18.

24. Krackow KA. *The Technique of Total Knee Arthroplasty*. St. Louis, Mo: The CV Mosby Company; 1990: Chap. 5, page 137.

25. Whiteside LA, Arima J. The anteroposterior axis for femoral rotation alignment in valgus total knee arthroplasty. *Clin Orthop*. 1995; 321: 168–172.

Chapter 3
Medial Release for Fixed-Varus Deformity

David J. Yasgur, Giles R. Scuderi, and John N. Insall

INTRODUCTION

Varus deformity of the knee is one of the most common deformities seen at the time of total knee arthroplasty. When a fixed deformity is present, the pathoanatomy usually involves erosion of medial tibial bone stock with medial tibial osteophyte formation, and contractures of the medial collateral ligament (MCL), posteromedial capsule, pes anserinus, and semimembranosus muscle (Fig. 3.1). Elongation of the lateral collateral ligament is a late event. A flexion contracture may coexist, which is manifested by contractures of both posterior capsule and posterior cruciate ligament.

Success and longevity of total knee arthroplasty is predicated in part on achieving proper limb alignment of 5 to 10 degrees of valgus.[1] The limb should be corrected to this ideal alignment without regard to the contralateral alignment, because a varus deformity often exists bilaterally. Furthermore, the ideal alignment of the femoral component is 7 ± 2 degrees of valgus angulation, whereas that of the tibial component is 90 ± 2 degrees relative to the longitudinal axis of the tibia.[1]

The ideal alignment is achieved through soft tissue releases aimed at balancing the collateral ligaments, and by placing the components in the correct orientation. If the proper alignment is not achieved, or if the ligaments are inadequately balanced, the components will be overloaded medially and subjected to excessive stresses, which may result in the eventual failure of the arthroplasty via either component loosening or accelerated wear. Intraoperatively, it is imperative to reassess each step of the soft tissue release so as not to overcorrect the deformity and create valgus instability.

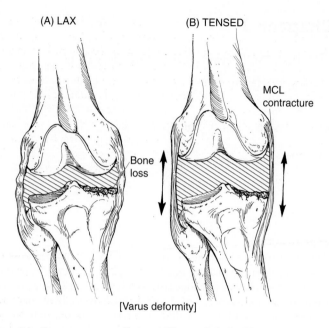

FIGURE 3.1. Genu varum usually caused by medial tibial bone loss and contractures of the medial soft tissue structures.

PREOPERATIVE PLANNING

A careful physical examination of the knee should assess the range of motion, flexion contracture, degree of deformity, ligamentous stability, and muscle strength. Anterior cruciate ligament deficiency is a common finding in a degenerative knee, but it is not a surgical dilemma in total knee arthroplasty. In contrast, deficiency of the posterior cruciate ligament (PCL) is much less common. A more likely scenario is the situation of a fixed-varus deformity with a flexion contracture, which requires resection of the PCL for complete correction of the limb alignment and flexion contracture. For these cases, a PCL-substituting design should be utilized. In those cases with severe contracture requiring extensive soft tissue release, a constrained condylar implant should be available. This is more often the case for severe genu valgum and not for fixed-varus deformities.

A detailed assessment of preoperative radiographs should be made for accurate preoperative assessment. This includes weight-bearing anteroposterior (AP), lateral, and tangential patella radiographs, as well as a full length standing AP radiograph. Patella tracking should be noted on the tangential patella view, because this may suggest preoperatively the need for lateral retinacular release. Bony defects should also be noted, because prosthetic augmentation or bone grafting may be required. The mechanical axis, degree of deformity, and femoral valgus should also be noted. If an intramedullary instrumentation system is utilized in which the valgus orientation of the distal femoral cut can be adjusted, then knowledge of the deformity and anatomic femoral valgus can allow one to slightly increase the valgus orientation of the distal femoral cut. This would then facilitate ligamentous balancing in severe fixed deformities.

TECHNIQUE

Approach

The anterior midline approach, with a medial parapatellar arthrotomy, is preferred because this allows for adequate exposure in most knees. It is also extensile in nature and can easily be converted into a quadriceps snip[2,3] or V-Y turndown[4] when warranted by knees that are difficult to expose, such as post-osteotomy or in patella infera. An anterior incision also allows for exposure of both medial and lateral supporting structures, and obviates the need for additional incisions.

The anterior longitudinal skin incision is carefully placed medial to the tibial tubercle to avoid a tender scar postoperatively. Following this, a medial parapatellar arthrotomy is carried out through a straight incision extending over the medial one-third of the patella and is continued onto the tibia 1 cm medial to the tibial tubercle. The quadriceps expansion is peeled off of the anterior patella via sharp dissection. The synovium is divided in line with the arthrotomy, and the anterior horn of the medial meniscus is divided. Patellofemoral ligaments are released, and the patella is everted and dislocated laterally, while the knee is flexed up.

The anterior cruciate ligament, if present, should then be divided, as should the anterior horn of the lateral meniscus, which will facilitate eversion of the extensor mechanism. To avoid avulsion of the tibial tubercle, the patellar tendon should be dissected subperiosteally with a cuff of periosteum to the crest of the tibial tubercle. As much as one-third of the tubercle may be exposed, but this is rarely necessary. Lastly, the fat pad and synovium can be resected to help expose the lateral tibial plateau. This exposure is the most versatile and utilitarian of all the exposures for total knee arthroplasty.

Medial Release

To correct a fixed-varus deformity, progressive release of the tight medial structures is performed until they reach the length of the lateral supporting structures.[3] The release is begun with the knee in extension using sharp dissection of a subperiosteal sleeve from the proximal anteromedial tibia (Fig. 3.2). A periosteal elevator is useful in continuing this dissection to the midline. Care should be taken to pass the elevator deep to the superficial MCL. The elevator should be used at a level approximately 3 to 4 cm from the medial tibial plateau, where the medial metaphysis is curving to join the tibial diaphysis. It is at this location where the inferomedial geniculate artery may be seen (Fig. 3.3). A bent Hohmann retractor may then be placed, being sure that the tip is deep to the

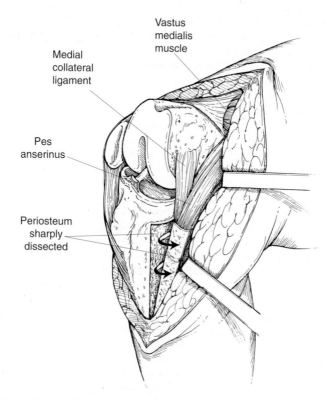

FIGURE 3.2. Subperiosteal sleeve sharply dissected from proximal anteromedial tibia, including superficial and deep MCL, along with the pes anserinus tendons, if needed.

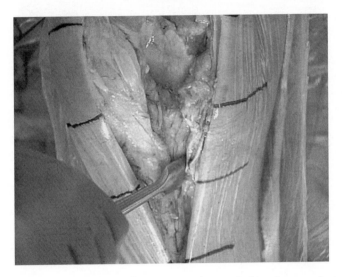

FIGURE 3.3. Subperiosteal sleeve continued posteriorly, using a periosteal elevator.

MCL (Fig. 3.4). Placement of this retractor allows for traction to be placed on the medial structures, thereby facilitating subperiosteal dissection.

With the knee in extension, a flat three-fourths inch osteotome is passed distally and deep to the superfical MCL (Fig. 3.5). A complete release requires that the osteotome be passed as much as 6 inches distal to the medial tibial plateau. Depending on the degree of release required, the pes anserinus can also be completely detached, or left partially attached as the osteotome elevates the MCL immediately posterior to the most anterior attachment of the pes tendons. Similarly, the osteotome can be used to release the deep attachment of the soleus muscle from the posteromedial tibial metadiaphysis.

Sharp dissection can then proceed superiorly to the level of the joint, which will elevate the deep MCL off of the tibia. Proceeding posteromedially with the lower leg externally rotated and the knee flexed, one can sharply elevate the semimembranosus off of the tibia, which often liberates fluid from the semimembranosus bursa

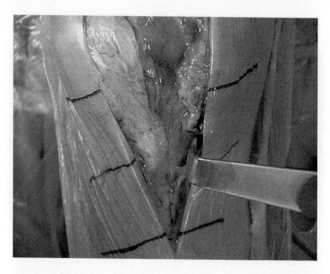

FIGURE 3.4. Hohmann retractor placed deep to subperiosteal sleeve places tension on structures, permitting further dissection.

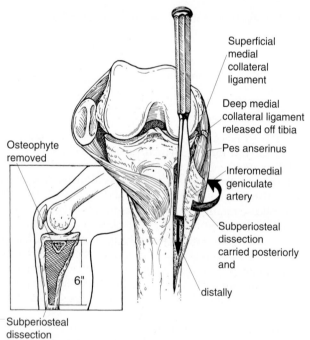

Superficial medial collateral ligament

Deep medial collateral ligament released off tibia

Pes anserinus

Inferomedial geniculate artery

Subperiosteal dissection carried posteriorly and

distally

Osteophyte removed

6"

Subperiosteal dissection

FIGURE 3.5. Osteotome inserted deep to periosteal flap or MCL, used to subperiosteally strip medial supporting structures from proximal tibia, while maintaining a continuous soft tissue sleeve.

(Fig. 3.6). In this way, the posteromedial tibia can be safely exposed to the midline. At this point, the tibia appears skeletonized (Fig. 3.7). Medial tibial osteophytes may serve to tighten the medial side, because the MCL is draped over the osteophytes. Thus, resection of the medial tibial osteophytes is the final step in releasing a fixed-varus knee. It is often useful to wait until a trial tibial component has been inserted before resecting the medial tibial osteophyte. In that way, one can use the trial component as a template and ensure that excessive bone is not excised.

Over release of the medial structures in a knee with even a mild deformity is usually not encountered, because this technique ensures that the MCL is not transected, but rather is maintained as a continuous sheet of tissue confluent with the periosteum. The extent of release can be monitored by placing the knee into full extension and exerting a valgus force. Alternatively, lamina spreaders can be gently inserted into the femorotibial articulation (Fig. 3.8) and the alignment judged with a plumb line.

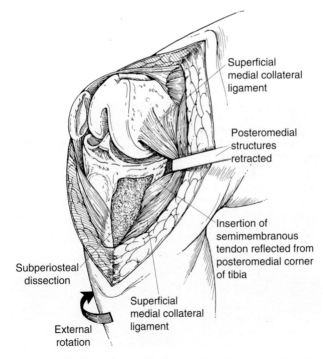

FIGURE 3.6. Semimembranosus insertion sharply dissected with tibia externally rotated.

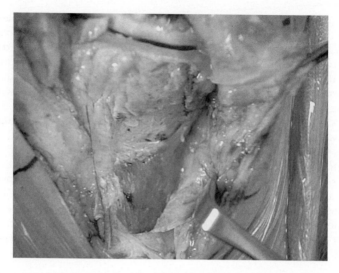

FIGURE 3.7. Skeletonized appearance of tibia after semimembranosus released.

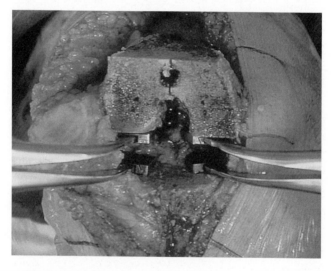

FIGURE 3.8. Laminar spreaders are useful in monitoring soft tissue balance and ligament releases.

The cruciate ligaments may inhibit correction and should then be resected. Attempts to retain the PCL in cases of severe varus deformity usually result in failure to adequately correct the deformity. Although it is attractive to some to progressively release the PCL and use a cruciate-retaining (CR) type of prosthesis, we prefer to sacrifice the PCL and use a posterior cruciate-substituting prosthesis. Furthermore, literature suggests that the PCL is often non-functional in CR knees, as evidenced by anterior translation of the femur on the tibia, or "rollforward."[3,5] Besides limiting correction, retention of a tight PCL can limit motion. In this case, the knee may fail to have the gliding and rolling that occurs with flexion and may open anteriorly like a book during flexion. Such phenomenon may account for component loosening in CR knees.[3]

When the medial release has been completed and proper alignment has been achieved, the standard bone cuts are then made. The distal femur is cut first with an intramedullary instrument that allows variation of the valgus orientation of the femoral component. For severe varus deformities, one may want to slightly increase the valgus orientation of the distal femoral cut to help facilitate soft tissue balancing. The femur is then sized and the appropriate cutting block is selected. The anterior and posterior surfaces of the femur are then cut with instrumentation that is rotationally aligned with the epicondylar axis[6,7] and that incorporates principles of anterior and posterior referencing into the same guide (Fig. 3.9). Care

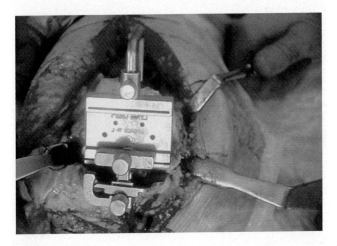

FIGURE 3.9. Anteroposterior femoral cutting guide is aligned along the epicondylar axis and incorporates principles of anterior and posterior referencing.

is taken to position this cutting guide so that the posterior condyles are not over- nor underresected, and that the femur is not notched anteriorly.

The remnants of the cruciate ligaments and menisci are then resected, as are the intercondylar osteophytes. Meticulous attention is then turned toward resection of posterior osteophytes because they may limit flexion. A curved three-fourths inch osteotome is used to resect this bone, as well as to perform a release of the posterior capsule off of the distal femur, when indicated (Fig. 3.10). This maneuver is particularly useful in correcting flexion contractures, but is also useful for releasing the medial gastrocnemius in knees with flexion contractures and fixed-varus deformities.

The tibial cut is then made utilizing an extramedullary guide adjusted to be perpendicular to the longitudinal axis of the tibial diaphysis, to match the posterior slope of the tibial plateau, and to resect approximately 1 cm of bone from the normal lateral tibial plateau. One should not resect the proximal tibia so as to eliminate any medial tibial bone defect that may exist, because this may be excessive.

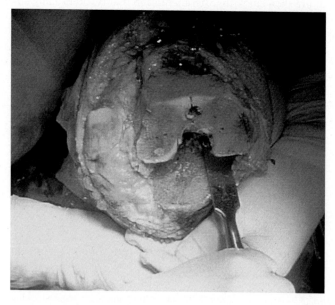

FIGURE 3.10. Curved osteotomes are used to remove posterior condylar osteophytes and recreate the posterior recess.

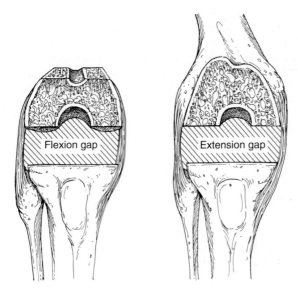

FIGURE 3.11. The flexion and extension gaps should be equal and rectangular in shape.

The ligament balancing, as well as the overall limb alignment, is then assessed with the use of spacer blocks in flexion and extension. When performed in this manner, with soft tissue release preceding bony resection, the flexion and extension gaps are rectangular and are usually equal in magnitude (Fig. 3.11). Occasionally, the extension gap may be tighter than the flexion gap, necessitating re-cutting of the distal femur to equalize the flexion-extension gaps.

Alignment of the femoral cutting block with the epicondylar axis[6,7] is a more precise way of ensuring that the femoral component is externally rotated. This also helps to balance the collateral ligaments in flexion. Excessive external rotation of the femoral component should be avoided, because this will result in an asymmetric flexion space. Additionally, internal rotation of either the tibial component or the femoral component is to be avoided, because patellar instability may result.

The management of tibial bone defects is beyond the scope of this chapter. One suggestion that has been worthwhile is lateralization of the tibial component, because this may reduce the need for augmentation of a medial tibial defect.

RESULTS

The technique described in this chapter for releasing the medial structures of the knee, balancing the ligaments, and restoring the normal alignment of the knee has proven to be successful. The survivorship data[8,9,10,11] and results of clinical and radiographic follow-up studies[1,12,13] have shown that this technique for medial release of fixed-varus deformities is both predictable and durable.

In a long-term follow-up of total condylar knees, the most senior author (JNI) and colleagues reported on 130 TKAs.[13] Of these, 63 (48%) had a varus deformity, including 23 (18%) who had a fixed-varus deformity of at least 10 degrees. At 10- to 12-years of follow-up, 88% had good to excellent results. Varus-valgus stability was maintained in all cases, except in one in which proper soft tissue balancing was not achieved, and varus instability recurred. In all, 81% had less than 5 degrees of instability to varus-valgus stress when tested in full extension.

Testing collateral stability in positions other than full extension is unreliable, because the lack of conformity in the prosthesis will allow some laxity with flexion. When the soft tissues are balanced meticulously, the released medial structures are usually not over-released, but rather remain contiguous with the medial tibial periosteum.

As stated earlier, it is our preference to sacrifice the cruciate ligaments and use a posterior cruciate-substituting prosthesis in correcting a fixed-varus deformity. Though it is our belief that PCL preservation may limit full correction of a fixed deformity, others have found that routine excision of the PCL is unnecessary, and that a CR knee can be used in cases of fixed-varus deformity.[14] Here, recession of the PCL must allow for correction of deformity, without creating posterior cruciate incompetence. This may be a formidable, if not impossible task, because fluoroscopic kinematic analysis of CR knees has demonstrated anterior sliding with flexion, secondary to PCL imbalance.[5]

COMPLICATIONS

Several complications can occur from the correction of fixed-varus deformities. These include instability of the tibiofemoral or patellofemoral articulations, or avulsion of the tibial tubercle.

Instability

Instability can occur in either extension or flexion, and can be either symmetric or asymmetric. Symmetric extension instability usually occurs from excessive resection of the distal femur, resulting in an extension gap that is inadequately filled by the components. Insertion of a thicker spacer may solve this problem, whereas creating a new one in that the flexion gap may now be too tight. A better solution is to build up the distal femur with the use of modular femoral augments.

Asymmetric extension instability is likely due to improper balancing of the collateral ligaments. This occurs when the contracted tight medial structures are inadequately released, or due to inadvertent division of the MCL. If the collateral ligaments cannot be balanced with soft tissue releases, or if the MCL is incompetent or transected, a constrained condylar implant may be needed.

Flexion instability may be asymmetric if the femoral component is malrotated into either internal rotation or excessive external rotation. Varus release balances the knee in extension, whereas external rotation of the femoral component creates a balanced, rectangular flexion gap. We prefer to set the rotational alignment of the femoral component along the epicondylar axis[6,7] to avoid excessive external rotation and internal rotation.

Symmetric flexion instability may paradoxically arise from insufficient resection of the distal femur. The tight extension gap then dictates a thin spacer, which inadequately fills the flexion gap, thereby creating flexion instability. The solution here would be to resect additional distal femur by an amount dictated by the difference in the thickness of the spacers used in flexion and extension (Fig. 3.12).

Downsizing may also create flexion instability because the posterior condyles are over-resected and replaced by a lesser amount of component (Fig. 3.12). In theory, a similar phenomenon may be encountered by instrumentation systems that rely on anterior referencing alone. The latest system of instruments that we use combines anterior and posterior referencing into the same guide as to minimize this dilemma.

Patellar Instability

Patellar instability more typically presents a challenge following correction of a fixed-valgus knee. However, even in a varus knee, attention to proper alignment and positioning principles is of paramount importance to ensure proper patellofemoral kinematics.

The femoral and tibial components must not be internally rotated, but rather externally rotated, as mentioned earlier. Internal rotation of the femoral component will create an asymmetric flexion space as mentioned earlier, but will also shift the lateral trochlea anteriomedially. This will increase the patellofemoral joint reaction force in a lateral vector, increasing the tendency for wear and/or subluxation. Internal rotation of the tibial component will

2. Garvin KL, Scuderi GR, Insall JN. Evolution of the quadriceps snip. *Clin Orthop.* 1995; 321:131–137.

3. Insall JN. Surgical techniques and instrumentation in total knee arthroplasty. In: Insall JN, ed. *Surgery of the Knee.* 2nd ed. New York: Churchill Livingstone; 1994: 739–804.

4. Trousdale RT, Hanssen AD, Rand JA, Cahalan TD. V-Y quadricepsplasty in total knee arthroplasty. *Clin Orthop.* 1993; 286:48–53.

5. Stiehl JB, Komistek RD, Dennis DA, Paxson RD, Hoff WA. Fluoroscopic analysis of kinematics after posterior-cruciate-retaining knee arthroplasty. *J Bone Joint Surg.* 1995; 77B:884–889.

6. Berger RA, Rubash HE, Seel MJ, Thompson WH, Crossett LS. Determining the rotational alignment of the femoral component in total knee arthroplasty using the epicondylar axis. *Clin Orthop.* 1993; 286:40–47.

7. Poilvache PL, Insall JN, Scuderi GR, Font-Rodriguez DE. Rotational landmarks and sizing of the distal femur in total knee arthroplasty. *Clin Orthop.* 1996; 331:35–46.

8. Colizza WA, Insall JN, Scuderi GR. The posterior stabilized total knee prosthesis. Assessment of polyethylene damage and osteolysis after a ten-year-minimum followup. *J Bone Joint Surg.* 1995; 77A:1713–1720.

9. Diduch DR, Insall JN, Scott WN, Scuderi GR, Font-Rodriguez D. Total knee replacement in young, active patients. Long-term follow-up and functional outcome. *J Bone Joint Surg.* 1997; 79A:575–582.

10. Scuderi GR, Insall JN, Windsor RE, Moran MC. Survivorship of cemented knee replacements. *J Bone Joint Surg.* 1989; 71B:798–803.

11. Stern SH, Insall JN. Posterior stabilized prosthesis. Results after follow-up of nine to twelve years. *J Bone Joint Surg.* 1992; 74A:980–986.

12. Insall JN, Hood JW, Flawn LB, Sullivan DJ. The total condylar knee prosthesis in gonarthrosis. A five- to nine-year follow-up of the first one hundred consecutive replacements. *J Bone Joint Surg.* 1983; 65A: 619–628.

13. Vince KG, Insall JN, Kelly MA. The total condylar prosthesis. Ten- to twelve-year results of a cemented knee replacement. *J Bone Joint Surg.* 1989; 71B:793–797.

14. Tenney SM, Krackow KA, Hungerford DS, Jones M. Primary total knee arthroplasty in patients with severe varus deformity. *Clin Orthop.* 1991; 273:19–31.

15. Scuderi G, Cuomo F, Scott WN. Lateral release and proximal realignment for patellar subluxation and dislocation. A long-term follow-up. *J Bone Joint Surg.* 1988; 70A:856–861.

16. Scuderi GR, Insall JN. Fixed varus and valgus deformities. In: Lotke PA, ed. *Knee Arthroplasty.* New York: Raven Press; 1995: 111–127.

17. Scuderi GR, Insall JN. Total knee arthroplasty. Current clinical perspectives. *Clin Orthop.* 1992; 276:26–32.

Chapter 4
Lateral Release for Fixed-Valgus Deformity

Frankie M. Griffin, Giles R. Scuderi, and John N. Insall

VALGUS DEFORMITY IN TOTAL KNEE ARTHROPLASTY

Fixed-valgus deformity of the arthritic knee can be a difficult and challenging problem in total knee arthroplasty. Varus deformity is more commonly encountered, and therefore most surgeons are more comfortable with the surgical principles and releases used on the medial side of the knee. At our institution, at the time of knee replacement we encounter fixed-varus deformity (50 to 55%) three times more frequently than fixed-valgus deformity (10 to 15%). Ligament balancing and changes in boney anatomy of the valgus knee may be more difficult to correct than with varus deformity. In addition, the correct sequence and technique of release of the lateral structures remain controversial. Many different techniques to correct valgus deformity have been described, and they demonstrate the lack of a consensus among surgeons. Potential complications—including peroneal nerve palsy, flexion or extension instability, and patellar maltracking—also make correction of valgus deformity challenging.

PATHOPHYSIOLOGY

The normal knee is aligned with a femorotibial angle of 6 to 7 degrees valgus, has a full range of motion, and may be slightly more lax laterally in flexion. In arthritis of the knee, loss of bone and cartilage leads to instability, which can be classified as either symmetric or asymmetric. In response to the instability, adaptive changes occur. In fixed-valgus deformity the instability is asymmetric, and the surgeon is faced with deficiency of the lateral bone and cartilage, contracture of the lateral ligaments and capsule, stretching of the medial ligaments, and contracture of the iliotibial tract. The structures that may be "tight" include the lateral capsule, lateral collateral ligament, arcuate ligament, popliteus tendon, lateral femoral periosteum, distal iliotibial band, and lateral intermuscular septum.[1] In addition, there may be asymmetric wear of the posterior condyles with excessive wear of the posterolateral condyle. This wear has implications in surgical technique if the posterior condyles are utilized to reference femoral component rotational alignment.[2] Some authors have also reported external rotation deformity of the proximal tibia due to the tight iliotibial tract.[3]

SURGICAL TECHNIQUES

Implant Selection

The successful results of total knee arthroplasty with the posterior-stabilized design are well documented in the literature.[4] In severe deformity, the PCL is often contracted and may limit correction of the deformity as described by Krackow's "cruciate limitation effect."[5] Even when an attempt at PCL-retention was made, Laurencian found that in 16% of knees he had to release the PCL.[6] Appropriate soft tissue balancing is much easier if the PCL is sacrificed. We believe it is much simpler to substitute a mechanical PCL for the diseased and contracted PCL in the severely deformed knee and that the results for the average surgeon will be better when the PCL is sacrificed routinely than when an attempt is made at soft tissue balancing with partial releases of the PCL and use of a posterior cruciate-retaining prosthesis. We therefore recommend use of the posterior-stabilized design.

In elderly low-demand patients, we prefer to use a constrained condylar knee to avoid the morbidity of extensive releases on the lateral side of the knee and to avoid the potential complications of peroneal nerve palsy and instability in flexion or extension. Bullek and associates (1996) evaluated the results of index-constrained condylar total knee arthroplasty in 28 patients with 34 TKAs.[7] The average age was 74.5 years, and the average preoperative deformity was 22 degrees valgus. No attempt at soft tissue balancing with lateral releases was made. Sixty-two percent required lateral retinacular releases for patellar tracking. All 34 TKAs (100%) had excellent (25 knees) or good (9 knees) results at an average follow-up of 3 years, and there was no evidence of early loosening or osteolysis. In younger patients, every attempt should be made to balance the knee and to avoid use of the constrained implant to eliminate the concern of early loosening in the more active, younger population.[8]

In some cases with bone deficiency, a modular implant with metal augments, offset stems, and variable tibial polyethelene thicknesses may be useful. In valgus deformity, patellar tracking is almost always an issue with lateral release rates reported from 62 to 100%.[7,8] Though one may speculate that the use of an implant

TABLE 4.1. Sequences of release

Author	First step	Second step	Third step	Final steps
Insall[17,18]	Posterolateral corner	Iliotibial tract	LCL, LIS	CCK
Ranawat[21]	Iliotibial tract transverse (2.5 cm)	Popliteus, LCL	Posterior capsule	LIS, lateral head of gastrocnemius
Keblish[10]	Lateral approach	Iliotibial tract multiple puncture	Posterolateral corner	Gerdy's tubercle, tibial tubercle elevation
Buechel[13]	Lateral approach	Iliotibial tract	LCL, popliteus	Fibular head excision
Clayton[14]	LCL, popliteus, lateral capsule	Posterolateral capsule, lateral head gastrocnemius, LIS	Iliotibial tract	Biceps femoris tendon Z-lengthening
Whitesides[3]	Iliotibial tract	Popliteus	LCL	Lateral head of gastrocnemius
Krackow[20]	Iliotibial tract	Popliteus	Posterolateral capsule, popliteus	Biceps femoris tendon, lateral head of gastrocnemius, MCL advancement in Type II

LIS = Lateral intermuscular septum
LCL = Lateral collateral ligament
CCK = Constrained condylar knee

visualization from inside to out (Fig. 4.4). It is helpful to keep the laminar spreaders in place during this release and to periodically squeeze them to stretch the lateral side. This works like a tensor and allows the lateral tissues to lengthen and slide with some degree of continuity. The incisions begin at the level of the joint line and are usually taken to a level approximately 10cm proximal to the joint line. The release is carried further proximally if necessary. By this stage, a "pop" is usually felt and the valgus deformity is adequately corrected. The popliteus tendon should be preserved if possible to provide lateral stability in flexion. In our hands, release of the ITB and posterolateral corner corrects the majority of fixedvalgus deformities. If further release is still necessary, we proceed with a subperiosteal release of the remaining lateral structures including the lateral intermuscular septum to a point 7 to 8cm from the joint line so that the whole "flap" is free to slide (Fig. 4.5). By this stage, almost all cases will have balanced, but if in the rare case further release is needed, we would release the lateral head of the gastrocnemius from its femoral attachment. Release of the biceps femoris should be avoided if at all possible. If after complete release the medial ligament is too lax, then the ligament

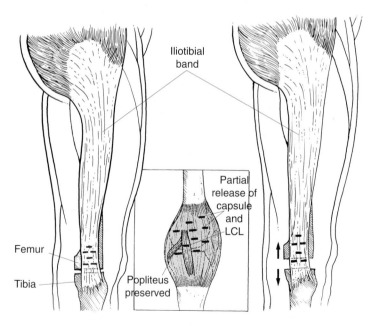

FIGURE 4.4. Piecrusting technique for valgus deformity.

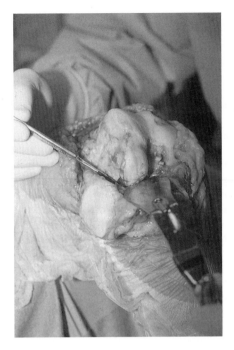

FIGURE 4.5. Lateral release from the distal femur for extreme valgus deformity.

reconstruction procedures described by Krackow[5,20] should be considered, although we have limited experience with this option. Finally, if ligament stability cannot be achieved, a constrained condylar implant will be used.

Patellar maltracking is often associated with a valgus deformity. If present, a lateral retinacular release should be performed.

Postoperative Management

Patients who have undergone ligament releases for fixed-valgus deformity are managed in a manner similar to those who have had routine total knee arthroplasties. The knee is placed in a continuous passive motion (CPM) machine in the recovery room, because we have found CPM to decrease the rehabilitation period required to achieve 90 degrees of flexion.[22] To avoid a postoperative flexion contracture, we recommend use of a knee immobilizer during sleep for patients who have a tendency to flex their knee while sleeping. On the second postoperative day, patients are instructed to stand with assistance, and by the third postoperative day, they resume walking with full weight-bearing with crutches or a walker. Goals for hospital discharge include independent ambulation with crutches or a cane, ability to climb stairs, and attainment of 90 degrees of flexion.

COMPLICATIONS

Peroneal Nerve Palsy

With release of the lateral structures and correction of valgus deformity, some stretching of the peroneal nerve is unavoidable and some degree of postoperative ischemia can be predicted with this stretching. Peroneal nerve palsy has been reported in 3% of patients who underwent TKA with preoperative valgus deformity.[8] In addition to valgus deformity, risk factors that have been shown to increase the risk of peroneal nerve palsy include previous laminectomy and postoperative epidural anesthesia.[22] Some authors have described dissection of the peroneal nerve from its fascial sheath behind the fibular head and even fibular head resection in an attempt to avoid this complication.[10,13] However, a definitive benefit has not been shown and the possibility of direct injury is probably increased by the dissection. Therefore, we do not recommend direct exploration of the peroneal nerve. Idusuyi and associates (1996) reported that peroneal nerve palsy may present in a delayed fashion.[22] Placing the knee in a CPM machine in the recovery room reduces the tension on the peroneal nerve by allowing early flexion and by avoiding prolonged extension of the knee. If a peroneal nerve palsy is noted in the early postoperative period, the treatment is one of observation because the natural history of a postoperative peroneal nerve palsy is gradual partial or complete recovery. Stern and colleagues (1991) followed five patients with postoperative peroneal nerve palsies and noted that all tended to resolve over time, although all were left with some residual neurologic deficit.[8] Asp and Rand (1990) reported the natural history of 26 postoperative peroneal nerve palsies that occurred after 8998 TKAs.[23] In this group, they found that 18 had complete palsies and 8 had incomplete palsies with 23 combined motor and sensory deficits and 3 with only motor deficits. At an average of 5.1 years after TKA, 13 had complete recovery, 12 had partial recovery, and 1 had no improvement. Partial palsies had a better prognosis for complete recovery and had higher knee scores than those with complete palsies. Those with complete recovery also had higher knee scores than those whose recovery was incomplete. Krackow

geons cement all of the components with a single mix of cement. This technique can represent both a cost- and time-saving approach; however, it is much more demanding to set all of the components at once and does leave more possibility for malpositioning.

We presently use Simplex cement because the liquid, doughy, and final setup times are about the same. The patellar component is cemented at the same time as the femoral. The femoral cement is used in the doughy stage once the mixture is no longer "sticky." The patella is held in place in the bone bed with a clamp and the femoral component is impacted onto the distal femur with the cement placed on the exposed bone surface and with some cement placed on the posterior runners of the actual component. The posterior aspect of the femur is often obscured by the component itself and contact there is important. Therefore, we place cement on the runner itself to ensure full coverage. When the component is impacted onto the bone surface, there is a common tendency to place the component in the flexed position, especially because the cement covers the bone surface. The tendency is less common when the component design includes short condylar pegs; however, not all systems have the pegs. Thus, it is probably best to hand place the component onto the distal femur and adjust the early position before using mechanical impaction.

The two cement mixings are timed to allow for removal of the exposed cement from the femoral side without waiting for the complete setting of the cement. This usually requires a separation time of 2 to 3 minutes. It is important to observe the femoral side while turning direction to the tibial side to ensure that the femoral component does not lift off during the final setup stage and that it is not pulled off the bone surface in an overzealous attempt to expose the tibia for the cementing.

The tibial side is cemented last when a posterior-stabilized component is used. We prefer that this cement is slightly more liquid to allow for better penetration into the proximal tibia. The cement is hand applied and the intramedullary peg hole is manually "pressurized" with thumb pressure to block off the upper hole and force the cement into the metaphyseal bone. This technique develops a cement "bulge" about the distal intramedullary stem. The chief criticism of the "pressurization" technique for the tibial stem is the greater difficulty of removal of the complex with an increase in loss of bone substance. The author has performed approximately 1000 arthroplasties with this technique and has had 3 tibial loosenings (in the same series we have about 6 femoral loosenings). Less than

5 tibial components have required removal because of infection, and no significant bone compromise has occurred with the extraction of the tibial tray and the cement. The author does, however, agree that the technique for tibial component cementing remains controversial.

After the excess peripheral cement is removed from the tibial tray, the knee is located and extended with slight manual pressure to compress the components onto the bony surfaces. When the bone is osteoporotic (such as in the rheumatoid knee), the extension maneuver should be performed with care to avoid collapse of the underlying bone and loss of fixation of the components. We again remove excess cement before it is completely set up and hold tourniquet release until the cement is solid in order to preserve the bone-cement interface.

Our technique is individualized to our own prosthetic line and prosthetic design. At the present time in the United States there are more cruciate-retaining total knees performed than posterior-stabilized. The cruciate-retaining knees are often performed as "hybrid" replacements. The tibial and patellar components are cemented first, and the femoral component is impacted onto the distal femur with a cementless design. This technique requires only one portion of cement but also requires a slightly more expensive femoral component for cementless application. Thus, the cementless component does save some time but the cost benefit is questionable.

There are several variations for the cementing of the tibial component depending upon the design of the tibial tray. Some trays include a central intramedullary stem of 3 to 4cm in length. Most surgeons cement the undersurface, including the stem. However, European surgeons often cement the undersurface and leave the stem uncemented and without a special surface for ingrowth. The latter technique is not recommended by most designers but is at the decision of the operating surgeon. The short intramedullary stem is designed to share load with the surrounding metaphyseal bone and performs this function best, if there is some bone ingrowth or if there is a cement mantle around the stem to transfer load over to the bone. If the stem is cemented or fully coated for bone ingrowth, revision surgery will certainly be more difficult and will probably lead to greater bone loss. Yet, poor fixation leads to loosening and a certain revision.

Other trays are designed with four short pegs of approximately 10mm in width and length that can all be cemented with the undersurface of the tray. Some new designs are returning to the all-polyethylene tibial component because of cost concerns. In this setting the entire component should be cemented, including the short intramedullary stem.

SUMMARY

At the present time, total knee surgeons are still faced with the decision concerning the type of fixation that they will rely upon for knee arthroplasty. The two camps have well-established theories. Cementless fixation has long-term results that are equal to those of the cemented prostheses. Studies out to 15 years and now approaching 20 years clearly document reliable results.[27–30] The well-ingrown total knee should remain fixed for a lifetime with just the possibility of polyethylene wear as the only consequence. The major problem with the cementless technology is the early loosening. Almost all studies report a 1% incidence most commonly on the tibial side. The loosening may be the result of surgical failure to establish full, acceptable surface contact. If this is the case, improvement in surgical technique should help to decrease loosening rates. There are new cutting instruments (such as milling devices) and guides that may improve surgical accuracy and increase contact. However, the loosening can be a result of micromotion at the interface that may be unavoidable if one expects to move the joint early after surgery to maintain range of motion. In this scenario, loosening may represent a persistent problem.

The cemented prostheses also have an excellent longterm history with similar 15- to 20-year results. The early loosening rate is well below 1% and is a rare occurrence. However, there is the lingering question concerning ultimate failure of the cement mantles. Thus far, this ultimate failure rate has not presented itself at the 15- to 20-year mark. Some investigators believe that the failure is inevitable. However, the surgeon must presently choose between a well-known early loosening rate with the cementless design or a theoretical concern for the future that has not as yet presented itself as a significant problem.

In light of this discussion, the author remains dedicated to cement fixation with an open eye toward the improvement of the cementless technology.

References

1. Verneuil AS. Affection articular du genou. *Arch med.* 1863.
2. Baer WS. Arthroplasty with the aid of animal membrane. *Am J Orthop Surg.* 1918; 16:1–29, 171–199.
3. Campbell WC. Arthroplasty of the knee: Report of cases. *Am J Orthop Surg.* 1921; 19:430–434.

Chapter 7
Cementless Total Knee Arthroplasty

Aaron A. Hofmann and David F. Scott

INTRODUCTION

Cementless total knee arthroplasty presently enjoys a success rate equal to cemented designs. Clinical results of early cementless total knee replacements had both design and development problems,[1–3] similar to early cemented systems.[2,4] Some early cementless knee series had suboptimal results, especially with metal-backed patellas.[5–10] Likewise, just as cemented total knee designs and clinical results improved,[11,12] so too have the evolution and clinical results of cementless total knee replacements. Cemented and cementless total knee arthroplasty are similar in respect to requirements for alignment, ligament balancing, and precise bone cuts. In order to achieve durable fixation, cementless fixation may require greater surgical precision than cemented TKA, and is optimized by certain prosthetic design modifications. Cementless fixation may provide several advantages, especially for the younger and more active patient. With increasing life expectancy, a more durable interface would be desirable, especially if bone rather than fibrous tissue attachment could be reproducibly assured. If porous-coated stems and pegs are avoided in the majority of primary total knee replacements, potential future revisions are more bone-sparing.

A number of recent reports indicate that excellent results can be obtained with cementless total knee arthoplasty,[13–17] especially if design considerations are coordinated with surgical technique. The authors' 7- to 11-year experience demonstrates that primary cementless fixation in an appropriately selected patient group provides results comparable to cemented TKA with the advantage of conserving bone stock and eliminating the potential problems of methylmethacrylate fixation.[18]

CEMENTLESS IMPLANT DESIGN

There are several important design and surgical considerations for cementless total knee arthroplasty components. These include biological issues such as the type of coating utilized to promote bone ingrowth, the routine use of morselized autogenous bone chips, and careful patient selection. Other considerations include the geometry of the components, and their alignment and kinematics after implantation.

CEMENTLESS IMPLANT DESIGN: BIOLOGIC CONSIDERATIONS

Patient Selection
We treat a relatively young (average age of TKA patient: 64 years) and very active patient population with osteoarthritis or well-controlled rheumatoid arthritis, and consequently select almost 90% for cementless fixation. Older, sedentary patients with poor bone quality or major medical problems are selected for cemented fixation.

Porous Coating
Although some early designs included femoral components fabricated from treated titanium alloy with a titanium alloy-polyethylene articulation, most femoral components are now fabricated from cobalt chrome for improved polyethylene wear and resistance to third body wear. Our choice for the porous coating is commercially pure titanium sintered to a cobalt chrome alloy substrate. This has been shown to provide excellent bone ingrowth.[19] Our preference for the femoral component is a bimetal design, combining the superior wear properties of cobalt chrome with polyethylene, and the biocompatibility of titanium.[20] This coating has an average pore size of 400μm and a porosity of 55%, compared to a beaded surface porosity of about 35% regardless of bead size.

Porous-coated pegs and stems are avoided to minimize stress-shielding of the interface and improve bone preservation during revision. Porous-coated pegs may cause a starburst pattern of bone ingrowth, which stress shields the remaining interface and causes significant bone loss if revision is required.

Autogenous Bone Chips as a Biologic Cement
Analysis of the resected proximal tibia reveals that the cortical bone surface area is an average of 6% of the total tibial surface, and that cancellous bone accounts for 18% of the total area, with bone marrow space comprising 76% of the remaining surface area.[21] The implication is that some form of "cement" is required to increase the surface attachment between the tibial component and the resected cancellous bone, and thus eliminate loosening and subsidence and provide durable fixation. The authors advocate the

routine use of autograft cancellous bone chips[22-25] as a biologic "cement" to improve bone ingrowth by reconstructing the subchondral bone region creating a dense neocortex at the implant interface, and to increase the cancellous bone surface attachment of porous-coated tibial components to host bone.[24,25] The autologous bone chips are prepared using the patellar reaming instruments on the cut surface of the tibial wafer.

The use of morselized autogenous bone chips appears to enhance the fixation of cementless components. An experimental study was performed in which paired porous-coated devices were implanted with and without the addition of morselized autogenous bone chips into the contralateral medial femoral condyle of patients undergoing the first stage of bilateral total knee arthroplasty.[25] The devices were removed *en bloc* at the second total knee arthroplasty. Backscattered electron imaging revealed significantly more bone in the implant with autogenous bone chips. Tetracycline labeling demonstrated that this was living bone. In a postmortem retrieval study[23] of tibial components implanted with and without supplementary morselized autograft bone chips, the tibial components implanted with bone chips had a clear advantage in bone ingrowth and bone apposition to the porous-coated surface. Postmortem retrieval analysis of 10 porous-coated tibial components implanted with autograft cancellous bone chips revealed bone in contact with 64% of the porous-coated interface, and backscattered electron imaging revealed bone ingrowth within 8 to 22% of the porous coating by volume[24] (Fig. 7.1).

CEMENTLESS IMPLANT DESIGN: GEOMETRY

Femoral and Tibial Component Design

An anatomic design with near-normal kinematics is required for successful cementless total knee arthroplasty. Smooth pegs are preferred for all three components. If a tibial stem is required, it should also possess a nonporous surface. The femoral component is a bimetal design as discussed previously. A deep trochlear groove is desirable because it improves range of motion, and minimizes patellar subluxation or dislocation,[2] and prevents excess wear and load on the patellar component. It should be angled 6 degrees as in the normal distal femur for proper tracking. Adeep trochlear groove avoids functional shortening of the extensor mechanism seen in knee systems that have shallow grooves.[2]

The proximal tibia is 5 to 6 mm smaller on the lateral side than on the medial side.[26] An asymmetric replacement will provide the

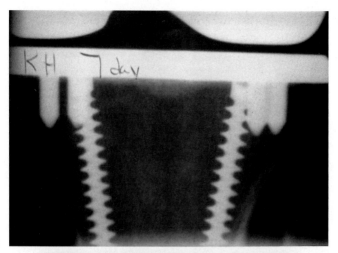

A

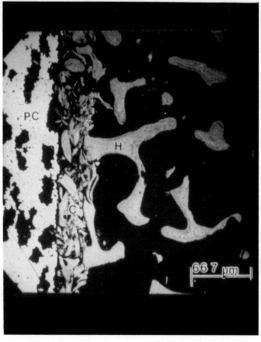

B

FIGURE 7.1. [A] "Blush" of bone chips immediately beneath tibial component 7-days postop. [B] Backscattered electron imaging showing the bone chips interposed between the porous coating (PC) and the host tissue (H). Three-week postmortem retrieval. [C] Tetracycline-labelled bone chips (BC) interposed between the porous coating (PC) and host bone (H) demonstrating viability and incorporation of bone chips at 12 weeks. Human in vivo plug model. [D] Bone ingrowth into retrieved tibial component 6-years postimplantation showing excellent bone ingrowth (B) into porous coating (PC). Osteointegration of bone and porpus coating demonstrated. Substrate (S).

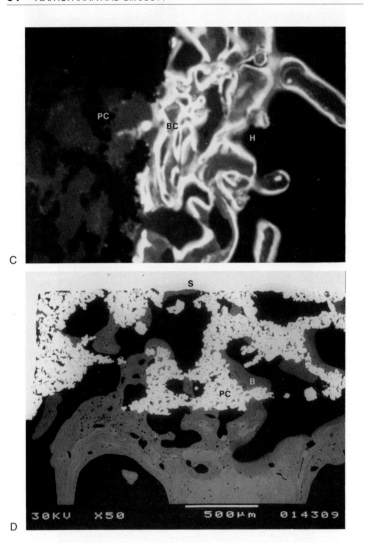

FIGURE 7.1. *Continued.*

best coverage of the proximal tibia and avoid soft tissue impingement. With symmetric replacements, the only options are undersizing the medial side or overhanging the lateral side.[27-29] It has been suggested that tibial coverage is inadequate with a symmetric tibial baseplate without overhang.[27,28] Tibial fixation and initial stability is also enhanced with two 6.5 mm titanium alloy cancel-lous bone screws that augment the components' four peripherally placed smooth pegs. A smooth central stem is recommended when fixation is required in softer bone (i.e., rheumatoid arthritic patients, osteoporotic females).[30]

Patellar Component Design

Failure of metal-backed patellar components has been attributed to insufficient polyethylene thickness around the periphery of the metal backing and the absence of an anatomically deep trochlear inset in the femoral component. Our preferred patellar compo-nent[31] has a modified dome-shaped polyethylene button that has a minimum 3 mm thickness around the periphery, and no overhang-ing polyethylene (Fig. 7.2). Patellar component fixation is aug-mented by three integral peripherally placed smooth pegs inserted into a planed flat bed. The thickness of the metal-backed patellar component can be accommodated without over-thickening the patella-implant complex by countersinking the implant 2 to 3 mm into the reamed bone bed. This is an essential surgical step in order to prevent the recent problems with metal-backed patellar components.

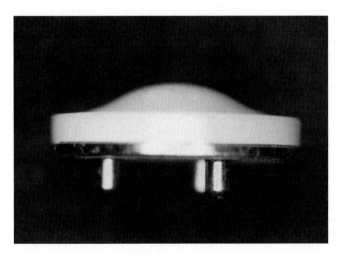

FIGURE 7.2. Photograph of metal-backed Natural-Knee™ patellar compo-nent demonstrating minimum 3 mm peripheral polyethylene thickness.

CEMENTLESS IMPLANT ALIGNMENT AND KINEMATICS

Restoration of Normal Alignment

Anatomic and radiographic studies reveal that the normal joint line is oriented horizontally. An average of 6 degrees of overall tibiofemoral valgus is produced by an average of 8 to 9 degrees of distal femoral valgus combined with an average of 2 to 3 degrees of proximal tibial varus (range: 0 to 6 degrees),[32] and the joint line is parallel to the floor. Following this orientation during total knee arthroplasty provides an anatomic alignment. This places the mechanical axis slightly into the medial compartment providing an even distribution of forces across an asymmetric tibial tray. No external rotation of the femoral component is required for this method.

Most total knee instrumentation produces a slightly different joint line, which is oriented perpendicular to the mechanical axis (from the center of the femoral head to the center of the ankle), due to a tibial resection that is perpendicular to the long axis of the tibia. The joint line produced is generally 2 to 3 degrees from parallel to the floor. Krakow has referred to this alignment approach as *classical* alignment.[33] Externally rotating the femoral component 3 degrees is recommended to compensate for the iatrogenic soft tissue imbalance that this creates (Fig. 7.3).

Our preference is to reestablish the normal anatomy as closely as possible, in order to achieve the goal of normal kinematics. Correct positioning of the implants is usually accomplished by cutting the tibia perpendicular for the valgus knee, or in slight varus in the frontal plane for the varus knee, and by cutting the distal femur in 6 degrees of valgus from the anatomic axis. This accomplishes an overall alignment of 4 to 6 degrees of valgus with better patellar tracking. A standard 6-degree valgus cut of the femur is recommended, although the instruments allow 4, 6, or 8 degrees. The anatomic-mechanical axis angle can be measured from a radiograph, but it may be inaccurate by 1 to 2 degrees because of rotational inconsistency. The true anatomic axis may be off with all intramedullary instruments if the starting point on the distal femur is too medial or lateral, or if the medullary rod is not perfectly centered in the medullary canal.

Restoration of Anatomy

A measured resection technique[33] is used for resurfacing the knee by referencing the least-diseased portion of the femoral condyle, the least-involved portion of the tibial plateau, and the thickest portion of the medial facet of the patella. The resected bone is

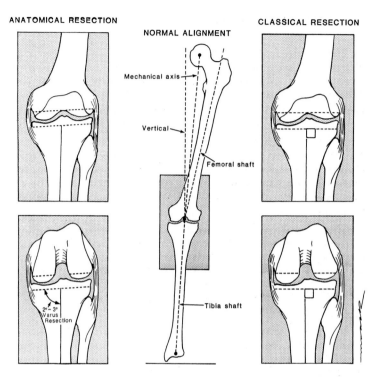

FIGURE 7.3. Anatomic and classical alignments. Note orientation of joint line with respect to floor.

replaced millimeter for millimeter with implant. This restores bony anatomy and the anatomic joint line. Knee rotation testing and computer modeling have shown that the level of resection relative to the amount replaced by the prosthesis on the distal femur plays an important role in knee kinematics and ligament balance. Resection of bone followed by an equal amount of prosthetic replacement will provide the knee with near normal varus-valgus and rotational stability throughout the full range of motion and excellent clinical results.

The level of the trochlear groove on the femur is anatomically restored by a stepped anterior chamfer cut that allows the bone to be resected and replaced with a deeply grooved femoral component. As a result, patellofemoral joint stability is achieved, making lateral release infrequent and, when required, less extensive. Increased patellofemoral compressive forces are avoided by maintaining the patellofemoral joint line, which reduces wear and patellar breakage and failure.

The tibial cut is made parallel to the joint line in the sagittal plane. Because the normal posterior tilt of the tibia is not at a fixed angle (range 4 to 12 degrees), this cut must be adjustable to reproduce each individual's normal posterior slope.[34] If the posterior slope is fixed at a single angle, the normal kinematics of the knee will not be simulated, because the PCL will be either too loose or too tight. Furthermore, cutting the tibia parallel to the patient's natural posterior slope greatly improves the load-carrying capacity of the supporting bone. A 40% improvement in ultimate compressive strength was noted when bone cuts were made parallel to the joint versus those made perpendicular to the tibial shaft axis.[34] Clinically, anterior subsidence is avoided if the tibial cut closely matches the anatomic posterior slope. Recent basic science investigations conducted in our research labs utilizing stereoscopic analysis have shown that when the bone is resected parallel to the natural anatomical slope, the trabeculae are oriented parallel to the resultant load.[35] This study provides a morphological explanation for the increased biomechanical strength measured in our previous study.[34]

For marked anatomic variation (i.e., malunion), an external alignment tower pointing toward the preoperatively marked femoral head can be utilized.

PCL Retention or Substitution
The authors argue that PCL retention better preserves the normal kinematics of the knee with maintenance of femoral rollback, clearance of the femur for increased range of motion and quadriceps strength, increased stair-climbing ability, fewer patellar complications, and reducing anteroposterior shear forces thus reducing bone-prosthesis interface shear stress.[36–41]

Balancing of the flexion and extension gaps is critically dependent upon the preoperative state of the posterior cruciate ligament. If the PCL is contracted in valgus knees or knees with fixed flexion deformities, flexion-extension balancing is difficult, and the PCL should be sacrificed. The PCL is often inadequate or absent in cases of inflammatory arthritis, as well as in some cases of advanced degenerative arthritis. When the PCL is sacrificed or incompetent, stability of the knee depends upon PCL substitution.[42–44] In traditional PCLsubstituting TKA systems, a central polyethylene post of the posterior middle portion of the tibial insert articulates with a transverse cam on the femoral component. As the knee flexes to 75 degrees, the post and cam come into contact, preventing the tibia from subluxating posteriorly and maintaining femoral rollback. Although this design has proven useful, it is not without problems and complications including post failure and dislocation. In order to improve results with posterior stabilization, a more congruent (ultracongruent) tibial polyethylene insert was designed[45] (Fig. 7.4). The insert is designed with an anterior buildup of 12.5 mm, and a more congruent articular surface to stabilize the femur in the anteroposterior plane, and has proven clinically successful for over 5 years.[45]

Patella Medialization

Patellar maltracking problems in total knee arthroplasty have ranged from 1 to 20% in the literature, and up to 50% of knee revisions are due to patella-related complications.[4,46,47] Multiple causes

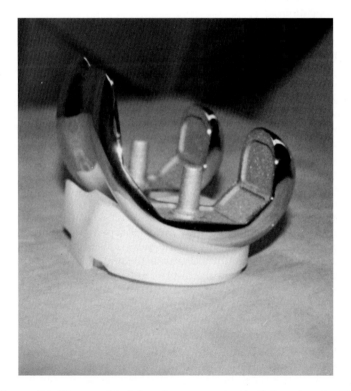

FIGURE 7.4. Photograph of the ultracongruent polyethylene insert with standard primary femoral component.

of patellar maltracking have been cited, including excessive post-operative valgus, internally rotated tibial or femoral components, malposition of the tibial or femoral component in the coronal plane, and malposition of the patellar component.[48-54] Correction of patellar maltracking has traditionally involved the use of a lateral retinacular release. Problems related to lateral retinacular release include increased postoperative pain and wound-healing complications, delayed rehabilitation, and compromised patellar blood supply.[15-17,19,27] Work at our institution has found that lateral retinacular release is required in 46% of patients whose patellar component is centralized on the patella, and in only 17% of patients whose patellar component is relatively medialized by centering over the anatomical high point or sagittal ridge.[55] This technique is described next in the techniques section. It must be emphasized that the previous design and combined surgical procedure, as mentioned before, must be followed to limit patellar complications.

SURGICAL TECHNIQUES

Surgical Approach

The subvastus approach is preferable for many total knee arthroplasties,[56] and is used by the senior author in 80% of cases. The subvastus approach should be avoided in situations that may make patellar eversion difficult, such as with previous lateral compartment scarring (tibial osteotomy), obesity, and patients with a prior medial arthrotomy. With a subvastus approach, the deep fascia of the thigh overlying the vastus medialis is incised in line with the skin incision. Using blunt dissection, this fascia is elevated off the vastus medialis obliquus (VMO). The inferior edge of the vastus is identified and lifted off the intermuscular septum using blunt dissection. The vastus medialis muscle belly is then lifted anteriorly. While under tension, the transverse tendinous insertion to the medial capsule is cut at the level of the midpatella, leaving the underlying synovium intact.

The arthrotomy is then performed vertically adjacent to the patella and the patellar tendon. The fat pad is incised at the medial edge to minimize bleeding and is not excised unless redundant. The patella is then carefully everted and dislocated as the knee is maximally flexed to provide generous exposure of the distal femur. If the patella is difficult to evert, a partial lateral release can be performed here for the heavy patient or the valgus leg with subluxating patella. The patella insertion device can be placed on the patella to facilitate eversion.

Preliminary proximal release of the tibial soft tissue is performed and should extend to the posteromedial corner of the tibia. All osteophytes are removed to identify true bony landmarks and dimension. If a marked deformity is present, further soft tissue release may need to be performed prior to making the bone cuts. However, this can usually be best titrated once the trials are in place.

Bone Cuts

Bone resorption and connective tissue formation occur when bone is surgically traumatized and heated to above 47°C for longer than one minute.[57] To control thermal injury, the sawblade is cooled by constant irrigation when making bone cuts. Without irrigation, any sawing or drilling can quickly raise the temperature of the bone to 170°C. All bone cuts should be made with a new sawblade coupled with a precisely toleranced saw capture. Sharp sawblades will decrease both operating time as well as trauma to the bone.

To ensure that a near perfect flat surface has been created, the saw capture is removed and all bone cuts sighted (in two planes) against the cutting blocks. Acentral high spot near the intercondylar notch of the femur may persist and will require additional planing. The high spot must be eliminated to keep the femoral component from becoming "high centered" when it is implanted. The high spot is eliminated by making a few extra passes with the sawblade using a slight upward spring of the blade against the bone. The flatness can also be checked using an auxiliary cutting block.

PCL Preservation

To preserve the PCL, it can be recessed 8 to 9 mm using a small knife blade, and protected by placing a small one-fourth-inch osteotome just anterior and deep to the ligament, preventing the sawblade from going too posterior.

Measured Resection Technique

Proper positioning of the joint line is essential for normal kinematics. The distal femoral alignment guide is applied and further stabilized by dialing the medial or lateral adjustable screw down to the defective distal femoral condyle. If both condyles are defective (i.e., with rheumatoid arthritis), both adjustable screws are dialed down slightly to compensate for the lost cartilage (2 to 3 mm). This maneuver avoids elevation of the joint line.

If the patient has normal proximal tibial varus, which ranges from 0 to 6 degrees,[32] it is preferable to make a 2-degree varus cut to allow resection of a more symmetrical wedge of proximal tibia. This will significantly improve soft tissue balancing and allow for proper orientation of the joint line. A caliper is used to measure the resected tibia in areas of relatively normal cartilage. Adding 1 mm to this measurement for bone loss from the saw blade will predict the thickness of the tibial replacement.

Before making any bone cuts, the maximum thickness of the patella is determined using a caliper. The total patellar resection should equal the thickness of the patellar insert, except in cases of severe patellar wear. Increasing the overal thickness of the patella-prosthesis construct will increase the patellofemoral joint forces and cause tracking problems and excessive wear, necessitating a lateral release. For improved fixation of the patella, countersinking the 10 mm components 2 to 3 mm is a routine procedure in our clinical practice.

Tibial Sizing

The surgeon should select the largest size tibial baseplate that does not overhang. Medial overhang is a recognized source of pes bursitis[58] and should be avoided. Sizing of the tibia is optimized by the use of an asymmetric tibial tray to obtain maximum coverage of the resected bone surface.

Patella Medialization

Using a one-eighth-inch drill, the middle of the highest portion of the sagittal ridge of the patella is drilled perpendicular to the articular surface to a depth of approximately 12 mm. A patellar osteotomy is then made at the osteochondral junction, removing 7 mm of bone. The previously drilled hole is then identified, and used as the landmark for centering the patellar implant. This acts as a guide for proper medialization of the patella. The patellar sizer is then used to identify the correct size of patellar component that can be centered over the drill hole to reproduce the position of the patient's original high point, and allow a continuous rim of bone around the implant (Fig. 7.5). Eccentric placement of the patella 3 to 4 mm toward the medial facet utilizing this technique allows for better tracking and improved clinical results as discussed previously.

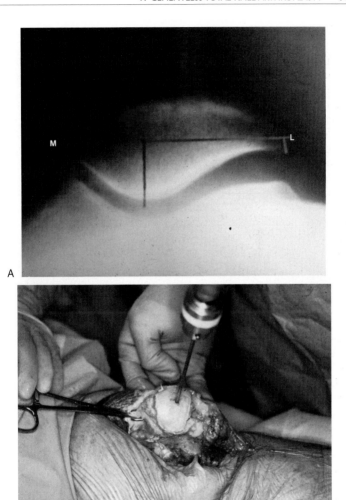

FIGURE 7.5. (A) Preoperative radiograph illustrating medial position of sagittal ridge of patella. (B) Drilling at the midpoint of sagittal ridge to mark the patella for medialization of the component. (C) Centering patellar reamer over the drill mark. (D) Postoperative radiograph of a medialized patellar component.

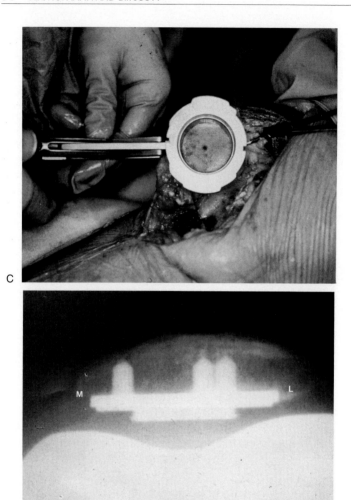

C

D

FIGURE 7.5. *Continued.*

Trial Reduction

Prior to trial reduction, posterior osteophytes on the femur are removed using a three-fourth-inch curved osteotome while lifting the femur with a bone hook. Osteophyte removal is essential for maximum knee flexion.

Stability is checked in full extension, 20 degrees of flexion, and full flexion. If the PCL is intact, slight medial and lateral laxity should be allowed. Full extension must be obtained on the operating table. The femur should track in the center of the tibial tray. If the PCL is absent, the next thicker size tibial insert must be selected. The slight flexion deformity this creates will stretch out over the first 6 months. It is suggested that the PCL be resected intentionally if the patient has more than 10 degrees varus or valgus deformity or more than a 10- to 15-degree flexion contracture preoperatively.

Implantation of Components-Morselized Autogenous Bone Grafting

A slurry of cancellous bone is obtained from the cut undersurface of the tibial wafer (Fig. 7.6). The patellar reamers are utilized for

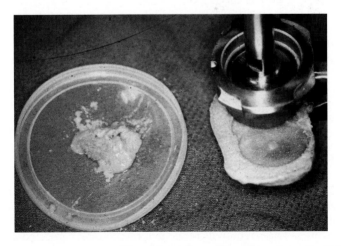

FIGURE 7.6. Preparation of bone slurry from the undersurface of a tibial wafer. Patellar reamer is shown reaming the undersurface of the resected tibial wafer. The autograft bone paste is seen in the plastic tray.

this purpose. This biologic bone "cement" is applied to every surface on the tibia, femur, and patella. In a routine varus knee, the bone is more porotic on the lateral side, and care is taken to spread additional bone slurry on the lateral tibial plateau to improve the contact between the implant porous coating and bone. This also serves to reinforce the bone in this region and rebuild the subchondral plate.

CLINICAL RESULTS

The early clinical results of cementless total knee arthroplasty were variable, with some reports not comparing favorably to the results of later cemented TKA designs.[1–3,59] However, with the development of instrumentation that allows precise bone preparation, and prostheses based upon sound biomechanical designs, the results of several different series of cementless TKA are now comparable to the best results of cemented TKA in the first 10 years of follow-up.

Whiteside[13] reported the 10-year survivorship analysis of a series of 265 cementless total knee components. One knee loosened during the 9- to 11-year follow-up period and was revised, and five knees were revised for infection. Five knees had revision of the patellar and tibial components for wear that began with the patella and later involved the tibia. Including infection as a mode of failure, the 10-year survivorship in this group was 94%. Ten years after surgery, 83.7% of the patients had no pain, 6.1% had mild pain, 8.2% had moderate pain, and 2% had severe pain. Knee flexion was 110 degrees preoperatively, and increased to 115 degrees at 2 years postoperatively and remained unchanged during the entire follow-up period.

Laskin[14] reported the 2-year results of 96 cementless total knee arthroplasties done using the Tricon-M prosthesis. Each patient was matched for age, body habitus, and diagnosis to a patient with a cemented total knee arthroplasty. There was no statistical difference between the two groups with respect to pain, range of motion, stability, or patient satisfaction.

Rosenburg and colleagues[15] reported the 3- to 6-year results of 132 cementless and 139 cemented Miller-Galante prostheses. The fixation technique was based on patient age, bone quality, and ability to delay full weight-bearing. Eight cemented knees and six cementless knees required component revision. No cemented knee failures were due to loosening, and two cementless knees were revised for tibial loosening.

Buechel and associates[60] reported the results of 147 cementless total knee arthroplasties with condylar femoral components, rotating metal-backed patellar components, and either meniscal-bearing or rotatingplatform tibial components. The 6-year survival rate of the bicruciate-retaining meniscal-bearing implant was 100%. The 6-year survival rate of the posterior cruciateretaining meniscal implant was 97.9%, and the 6-year survival rate of the rotating platform was 98.1%. In a second report of 80 cementless total knees of the above designs, 96.3% had a good to excellent clinical outcome at 12 years.[61]

The senior author (AAH)[31,62] has reported the 6- to 10-year results of cementless TKA. Between 1985 and 1989, 302 consecutive cementless posterior cruciatesparing TKAs were performed at the authors' institution. The implant used was the titanium alloy porouscoated Natural Knee™ (Intermedics Orthopedics, Inc. Austin, Texas). This implant system has a deep trochlear grooved femoral component with two smooth pegs and a metal-backed patella with three smooth pegs. The tibial tray is fixed with four smooth pegs and two fully threaded 6.5 mm cancellous screws. The tibial tray is asymmetrically designed to conform to the anatomy of the normal tibia, with the lateral side 4 mm smaller than the medial. At a 6- to 10-year follow-up, 59 patients had died and 31 were lost to follow-up, resulting in 212 knees available for long-term review. Radiographic evaluation obtained at each clinic v isit include fluoroscopically assisted views to allow for precise evaluation of the implant interface[63,64] (Fig. 7.7). The mean preoperative modified HSS knee score was 58, with a mean flexion of 105 degrees. Postoperatively, the mean HSS knee score plateaued at 99, and mean flexion was 122 degrees, excluding the scores of the patients requiring reoperation. There was no evidence of component subsidence or loosening requiring revision. There have been a total of 15 reoperations to date. Nine knees were revised for development of PCL insufficiency, necessitating polyethylene exchange to an ultracongruent insert. Two knees were revised for infection, and two were revised for tibial component oversizing. Nine patellar components were revised incidentally at the same time to a newer design metal-backed component with thicker polyethylene. Two revisions were specifically for patellar complications, one for maltracking and one for component wear. Overall component survivorship at 6- to 10-year follow-up is as follows: femoral component 98%, tibial component 98%, polyethylene tibial insert 95%, and metal-backed patellar component 96%.

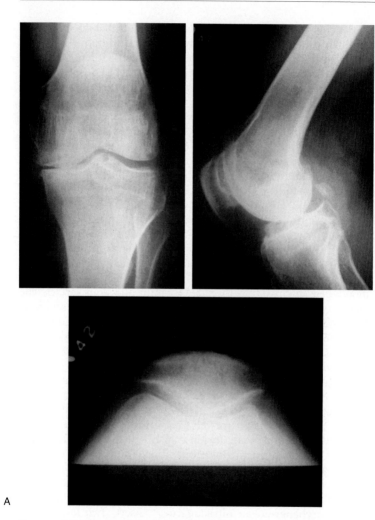

A

FIGURE 7.7. (A) Preoperative radiographs of a patient with varus osteoarthritis selected for cementless TKA. (B) Nine-year follow-up radiographs of cementless TKA revealing good position of components and no radiolucencies. Note preservation of polyethylene thickness of a patella component on skyline view, and tibial interface with an excellent bone apposition.

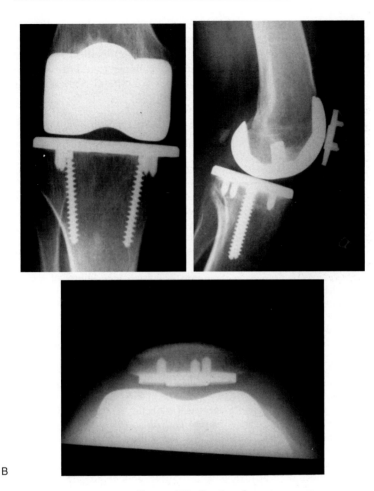

B

FIGURE 7.7. *Continued.*

CONCLUSIONS

Recent reports with up to 10-year clinical follow-up have demonstrated that cementless total knee arthroplasty can yield excellent results in young, active patients when sound implant design principles and surgical techniques are followed. Intimate apposition of the prosthesis to host bone is achieved with instrumentation that allows precise bone resection, and by the routine application of morselized autogenous bone chips to the cut surfaces. Revision of cementless total knee components without porous-coated pegs, keels, or stems has proven to be bone-sparing, which is an important consideration in the younger patient who may outlive their prosthesis. The authors believe that cementless fixation is a superior alternative to cemented fixation for primary total knee arthroplasty in younger patients with higher functional demands and good bone stock.

References

1. Hungerford DS, Krakow KA. Total joint arthroplasty of the knee. *Clin Orthop*. 1985; 192:23–33.
2. Moreland JR. Mechanisms of failure in total knee arthroplasty. *Clin Orthop*. 1988; 226:49–64.
3. Ranawat CS, Johanson NA, Rimnac CM, Wright TM, Schwartz RE. Retreival analysis of porous-coated components for total knee arthroplasty. A report of two cases. *Clin Orthop*. 1986; 209:244–248.
4. Insall JN, Hood RW, Flawn LB, Sullivan DJ. The total knee prosthesis in gonarthrosis. A five- to nine-year follow-up of the first one hundred consecutive replacements. *J Bone Joint Surg*. 1983; 65A:619–628.
5. Anderson H, Carsten E, Frandsen P. Polyethylene failure of metal-backed patellar components. *Acta Orthop Scand*. 1991; 62:1–3.
6. Baech J, Kofoed H. Failure of metal-backed patellar arthroplasty. *Acta Orthop Scand*. 1991; 62:166–168.
7. Bayley JC, Scott R, Ewald F, Holmes G. Failure of the metal-backed patellar component after total knee replacement. *J Bone Joint Surg*. 1988; 70-A:668–673.
8. Lombardi A, Engh G, Volz R, Albrigo J. Fracture/dissociation of the polyethylene in metal-backed patellar components in total knee arthroplasty. *J Bone Joint Surg*. 1988; 70-A:675–679.
9. Rosenberg A, Andriacci T, Barden R, Galante JO. Patellar component failure in total knee arthroplasty. *Clin Orthop*. 1988; 236:106–114.
10. Stulberg D, Stulberg B, Hamati Y, Tsao A. Failure mechanisms of metal-backed patellar components. *Clin Orthop*. 1988; 236:88–105.
11. Davies JP, Jasty M, O'Conner DO, Burke DW, Harrigan TP, Harris WH. The effect of centrifuging bone cement. *J Bone Joint Surg*. 1989; 71B:39–42.
12. Miller J. Fixation in total knee arthroplasty. In: Insall J, ed. *Surgery of the Knee*. New York: Churchill Livingstone; 1984:717–728.
13. Whiteside LA. Cementless total knee replacement. Nineto eleven-year results and 10-year survivorship analysis. *Clin Orthop*. 1994; 309: 185–192.
14. Laskin RS. Tricon-M uncemented total knee arthroplasty. A review of 96 cases followed for longer than two years. *J Arthroplasty*. 1988; 3: 27–38.
15. Rosenberg AG, Barden RM, Galante JO. Cemented and ingrowth fixation of the Miller-Galante prosthesis. Clinical and roentgenographic comparison after three- to six-year follow-up studies. *Clin Orthop*. 1990; 260:71–79.

16. Mont MA, Mathur SK, Krakow KA, Loewy JW, Hungerford DS. Cementless total knee arthroplasty in obese patients. A comparison with a matched control group. *J Arthroplasty*. 1996; 11:153–156.

17. Whiteside LA. Fixation for primary total knee arthroplasty: cementless. *J Arthroplasty*. 1996; 11:125–127.

18. Jones LC, Hungerford DS. Cement disease. [Review]. *Clinical Orthopaedics & Related Research*. 1987; 225:192–206.

19. Leland RH, Hofmann AA, Bachus KN, Bloebaum RD. Biocompatibility and bone response of human osteoarthritic cancellous bone to a titanium porous-coated cobalt chromium cylinder. *Transactions of the Society for Biomaterials*. 1991; 14:153 (abstract).

20. Hofmann AA. Response of human cancellous bone to identically structured commercially pure titanium and cobalt chromium alloy porous coated cylinders. *Clin Mater*. 1993; 14:101–115.

21. Bloebaum RD, Bachus KN, Mitchell W, Hoffman G, Hofmann AA. Analysis of the bone surface area in resected tibia. Implications in tibial component subsidence and fixation. *Clin Orthop*. 1994; 309:2–10.

22. Bloebaum RD, Bachus KN, Momberger NG, Hofmann AA. Mineral apposition rates of human cancellous bone at the interface of porous coated implants. *J Biomed Mater Res*. 1994; 28:537–544.

23. Bloebaum RD, Rhodes DM, Rubman MH, Hofmann AA. Bilateral tibial components of different cementless designs and materials: microradiographic, backscattered imaging, and histologic analysis. *Clin Orthop*. 1991; 268:179–187.

24. Bloebaum RD, Rubman MH, Hofmann AA. Bone ingrowth into porous-coated tibial components implanted with autograft bone chips: analysis of ten consecutively retrieved implants. *J Arthroplasty*. 1992; 7: 483–493.

25. Hofmann AA, Bloebaum RD, Rubman MH, Bachus KN, Plaster R. Microscopic analysis of autograft bone applied at the interface of porous-coated devices in human cancellous bone. *Int Orthop*. 1992; 16:349–358.

26. Krug WH, Johnson JA, Souaid DJ, Miller JE, Ahmed AM. Anthropomorphic studies of the proximal tibia and their relationship to the design of knee implants. *Trans Orthop Res Soc*. 1983; 8:402 (abstract).

27. Branson PJ, Steege J, Wixson RL, Stulberg SD. Rigidity of initial fixation in noncemented total knee tibial components. *Trans Orthop Res Soc*. 1987; 12:293 (abstract).

28. Dupont JA, Weinstein AM, Townsend PR. Tibial plateau coverage in total knee replacement. Tenth Annual Meeting Society for Biomaterials 1984; Washington, DC (abstract).

29. Westrich GH, Haas SB, Insall JN, Frachie A. Resection specimen analysis of proximal tibial anatomy based on 100 total knee arthroplasty specimens. *J Arthroplasty*. 1995; 10:47–51.

30. Lee RW, Volz RG, Sheridan DC. The role of fixation and bone quality on the mechanical stability of tibial knee components. *Clin Orthop*. 1991; 273:177–183.

31. Evanich CJ, Tkach TK, von Glinski S, Camargo MP, Hofmann AA. Six to ten year experience using countersunk metal-backed patellae. *J Arthroplasty*. 1996; In Press.

32. Moreland JR, Bassett LW, Hanker GJ. Radiographic analysis of the axial alignment of the lower extremity. *J Bone Joint Surg*. 1987; 69-A: 745–749.

33. Krakow KA. *The Technique of Total Knee Arthroplasty*. St. Louis: C.V. Mosby; 1990:118–137.

34. Hofmann AA, Bachus KN, Wyatt RWB. Effect of the tibial cut on subsidence following total knee arthroplasty. *Clin Orthop*. 1991; 269:63–69.

35. Bachus KN, Harman MK, Bloebaum RD. Stereoscopic analysis of trabecular bone orientation in proximal human tibias. *Cells Mater*. 1992; 2:13–20.

36. Andriacchi TP, Galante JO, Rermier RW. The influence of total knee replacement design on walking and stair climbing. *J Bone Joint Surg*. 1982; 64-A:1328–1335.

37. Ewald FC, Jacobs MA, Miegel RE. Kinematic total knee replacement. *J Bone Joint Surg*. 1984; 66-A:1032–1040.

38. Kelman GJ, Biden EN, Wyatt MP, Ritter MA, Colwell CW. Gait laboratory analysis of a posterior cruciate-sparing total knee arthroplasty in stair ascent and descent. *Clin Orthop*. 1989; 248:21–25.

39. Ranawat CS, Hansraj KK. Effect of posterior cruciate sacrifice on durability of cement-bone interface. *Orthop Clin N Amer*. 1989; 20:63–69.

40. Dorr LD, Ochsner JL, Gronley J. Functional comparison of posterior cruciate-retained versus cruciate-sacrificed total knee arthroplasty. *Clin Orthop*. 1988; 236:36–43.

41. Shoji H, Wolf A, Packard S, Yoshino S. Cruciate-retained and excised total knee arthroplasty. *Clin Orthop*. 1994; 305:218–222.

42. Insall JN, Lachiewcz PF, Burstein AH. The posterior stabilized condylar prosthesis: a modification of the total condylar design. *J Bone Joint Surg*. 1982; 64-A:1317–1323.

43. Scott WN, Rubenstein M, Scuderi G. Results after knee replacement with a posterior cruciate-sparing prosthesis. *J Bone Joint Surg*. 1988; 70-A:1163–1173.

44. Scuderi GR, Insall JN. The posterior stabilized knee prosthesis. *Orthop Clin N Amer*. 1989; 20:71.

45. Hofmann AA, Tkach TK, Evanich CJ, Camargo MP. Posterior stabilization in total knee arthroplasty with use of an ultracongruent polyethylene insert. *Orthopedic Transactions*. 1996; (abstract).

46. Cameron HU, Federhow DM. The patella in total knee arthroplasty. *Clin Orthop*. 1982; 165:196–199.

47. Clayton ML, Thirpathy R. Patellar complications after total condylar arthroplasty. *Clin Orthop*. 1982; 170:152–155.

48. Brick GW, Scott RD. The patellofemoral component of total knee arthroplasty. *Clin Orthop*. 1988; 231:163–178.

49. Anouchi YS, Whiteside LA, Kaiser AD, Milliano MR. The effects of axial rotational alignment of the femoral component on knee stability and patellar tracking in total knee arthroplasty demonstrated on autopsy specimens. *Clin Orthop*. 1993; 287:170–177.

50. Briard JL, Hungerford DS. Patellofemoral instability in total knee arthroplasty. *J Arthroplasty*. 1989; S87–S97.
51. Grace JN, Rand JA. Patellar instability after total knee arthroplasty. *Clin Orthop*. 1988; 237:184–189.
52. Merkow RL, Soudry M, Insall JN. Patellar dislocation following total knee replacement. *J Bone Joint Surg*. 1985; 67-A:1321–1327.
53. Nagamine R, Whiteside LA, White JE, McCarthy DS. Patellar tracking after total knee arthroplasty: the effect of tibial tray malrotation and articular surface configuration. *Clin Orthop*. 1994; 304:263–271.
54. Rhoads DD, Noble PC, Reuben JD, Mahoney OM, Tullos HS. The effect of femoral component position on patellar tracking after total knee arthroplasty. *Clin Orthop*. 1990; 260:43.
55. Hofmann AA, Tkach TK, Evanich CJ, Camargo MP, Zhang Y. Patellar component medialization in total knee arthroplasty. *J Arthroplasty*. 1997; 12(5):155–160.
56. Hofmann AA, Plaster RL, Murdock LE. Subvastus (southern) approach for primary total knee arthroplasty. *Clin Orthop*. 1991; 269:70–77.
57. Krause WL. Temperature elevations in orthopaedic cutting operations. *J Biomech*. 1982; 15:267–275.
58. Scott RD, Santore RF. Unicompartmental replacement for osteoarthritis of the knee. *J Bone Joint Surg*. 1981; 63A:536–544.
59. Collins DN, Heim SA, Nelson CL, Smith P. Porous-coated anatomic total knee arthroplasty. A prospective analysis comparing cemented and cementless fixation. *Clin Orthop*. 1991; 267:128–136.
60. Buechel FF, Pappas MJ. Long-term survivorship analysis of cruciate-sparing versus cruciate-sacrificing knee prostheses using meniscal bearings. *Clin Orthop*. 1990; 260:162–169.
61. Beuchel FF. Cementless meniscal bearing knee arthroplasty: 7- to 12-year outcome analysis. *Orthopedics*. 1994; 17:833–836.
62. Tkach TK, Evanich CJ, Hofmann AA, Camargo MP, Zhang Y. Six to ten year follow-up with cementless fixation. *Orthopedic Transactions*. 1996; (abstract).
63. Magee FP, Weinstein AM. The effect of position on the detection of radiolucent lines beneath the tibial tray. *Trans Orthop Res Soc*. 1986; 11:357 (abstract).
64. Mintz AD, Pilkington CA, Dip T, Howie DW. A comparison of plain and fluoroscopically guided radiographs in the assessment of total knee arthroplasty. *J Bone Joint Surg*. 1989; 71A:1343–1347.

Chapter 8
Three-Step Technique for Revision Total Knee Arthroplasty

Kelly G. Vince and Daniel A. Oakes

INTRODUCTION

Revision knee arthroplasty surgery requires that order be restored to the chaos of failure. Once the failed components, cement, and useless weak bone have been removed from the knee, a gaping hole confronts the surgeon. The problems of stability, mobility, fixation, and the reconstruction of bone defects as well as restoration of an anatomic joint line all cry out for attention at once. There are undoubtedly a variety of approaches to the revision knee surgery. One thing is certain—an organized approach is essential or the reconstruction is doomed to failure (Fig. 8.1).

This chapter proposes three steps to the reconstruction of any knee regardless of the original cause of failure. The surgeon must (1) reestablish the tibial platform, (2) stabilize the knee in flexion, and (3) stabilize the knee in extension. These steps have been described previously[1-3] and are based upon the principles of knee arthroplasty surgery that were developed for the total condylar knee prosthesis by John Insall, Chit Ranawat, and Peter Walker at The Hospital for Special Surgery in New York in the early 1970s.[4,5] We have applied these concepts to revision knee surgery, expanding them to address the rigors of the failed knee and establishing an appropriate sequence. Faithful adherence to the proposed sequence of steps, building one stage upon the other leads to a successful revision knee arthroplasty (Table 8.1).

Although contemporary instruments have enabled every surgeon to produce good primary knee arthroplasties, they rely on bone for reference. This bone simply does not exist in the failed knee. Consequently, instrument systems have not been reliable for revision surgery. Missing bone, however, is not the greatest challenge facing the surgeon. More problematic are the soft tissues. Working with strong concepts and trial components, the surgeon will be able to understand the vagaries of lost, plastically deformed, overly tight, and unreleased ligaments.

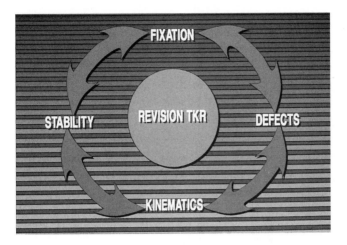

FIGURE 8.1. Diagram of problems of revision surgery.

This chapter does not deal with the diagnosis of a failed knee arthroplasty nor with the techniques for the removal of components from a failed knee. It must be emphasized, however, that no revision surgery should be attempted until an accurate mechanical explanation for the failure has been established. Revision of the inexplicably painful knee arthroplasty will yield miserable results.

Step 1 Establish Tibial Platform (Figure 8.2)
The tibia is a platform on which to rebuild the knee. The tibial articular surface is involved with knee function, irrespective of joint position. Whereas the distal femur bears load only in full extension and the posterior femur only in flexion, the tibia is constantly part of the articulation. The phrase tibial "platform" is chosen purposefully. Do not be concerned about the articular surface at this stage, that will come later.

The proximal tibia will have suffered any amount of insult from the failed joint. Although good-quality host bone is respected, any tibial cutting guide can be used to "square up" the surface by removing obviously weak and dispensable tissue. Defects are identified at this point, not eliminated. Any bone cut made now must not sacrifice good bone in an effort to eliminate a bone defect.

In many revision knee arthroplasties, medullary fixation will be required to enhance fixation. If so, open the medullary canal and confirm the measurements of endosteal diameter made on preoperative radiographs, using hand reamers. Bone should not be

TABLE 8.1. Three-step revision knee arthroplasty

Step	Goal	Key
1	Establish tibial platform	Tibia is common to flexion and extension gaps. It is a foundation to build on.
2	Stabilize knee in flexion	Femoral component size and position stabilize the knee in flexion.
2(A)	Sizing the femoral component	Do not simply fit component to the residual bone.
2(B)	Femoral component rotation	The component must not be internally rotated. Feel the residual posterior condylar bone as a guide. Use posterior lateral augments to correct internal rotation.
2(C)	Joint line	In general, a smaller femoral component leads to a higher joint line.
Decision 1	Gap mismatch	Flexion gap is so large due to soft tissue failure that the knee cannot be stabilized in flexion by the size of the femoral component. Need constrained component or ligament reconstruction.
3	Stabilize knee in extension	Seat the femoral component more proximally or distally to create an extension gap that equals the flexion gap.
Decision 2	Varus-valgus instability	The collateral ligaments are incompetent and either a constrained component or a ligament reconstruction will be required.

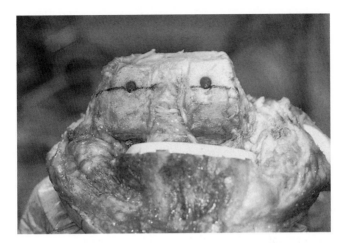

FIGURE 8.2. The tibial platform is reestablished.

removed from the tibial canal, which has a relatively thin cortex. A suitable trial rod is selected and attached to a trial tibial component. Once seated in the medullary canal, the tibial trial defines the defective bone that will require re-construction. If the intramedullary rod, fitted into the canal, is not parallel to the long axis of the tibia, the rod may be too wide for the asymmetric canal and either a narrower rod or one that is offset may be required.

There are several complex classification systems for describing bone defects at revision knee surgery. The simplest approach, in the course of a demanding surgery, will be the most helpful. Defects that are contained and have a rim of bone to hold bone graft, can be filled with particulate graft, be it autograft from the knee, ground up fresh-frozen bone, or freeze-dried allograft bone chips. Noncontained defects, as seen when a tibial component has sub-sided into varus, will most easily be dealt with by modular wedges or blocks. Combined contained and noncontained defects exist and respond well to a combined approach—the contained area is filled with graft and the noncontained area is reconstructed with an augment on top of the graft (Table 8.2).

Massive defects that offer virtually no host bone on which to seat any of the component will usually require reconstruction with structural allograft. These unusual situations should still be reconstructed following the three steps that are described here.

TABLE 8.2. A simple approach to bone defects

Bone defect	Solution
Contained	Particulate bone graft
Noncontained	Modular wedge or block
Massive	Structural allograft

Tibial defects can be reconstructed at this stage and the tibial component even cemented into place to save time. This is because the tibial platform does not affect how we reestablish alignment, stability, and motion in the knee. We build the knee upon the tibia. Tension and laxity in flexion and extension are manipulated with the femoral component. Nonetheless, in the interest of keeping most of our options open, it is best to leave the trial tibia in place, noting the type of bone defect if any and how we plan to reconstruct it when we implant the final components.

Step 2 Stabilize Knee in Flexion (Figure 8.3)

(A) Choose the Size of the Femoral Component That Stabilizes the Knee in Flexion

Choose the size of the femoral component that stabilizes the knee in flexion. It is a common and deadly error to measure existing bone and simply fit the corresponding femoral component to it. In almost every case, this will lead to the selection of a femoral component that is too small and an arthroplasty that is unstable in flexion or one in which excessive distal femoral bone must be resected to accommodate an unduly thick articular polyethylene. Undue resection of distal femur results in an unacceptable proximal migration of the joint line.

Ignore the residual bone on the distal femur in this step and visualize the normal bone that was present before any surgery had been performed. Use the size of the failed component, and lateral radiographs of the contralateral knee, if unoperated, to estimate the size of the revision femoral component. The final choice of revision femoral component size will depend upon the anteroposterior dimension that is necessary to stabilize the knee in flexion. The revision femoral component size will be determined not by residual bone, so much as by the soft tissues, specifically the collateral ligaments.

Stability in flexion is determined not only by the size, but also by the anteroposterior location of the femoral component. Unless the original component was oversized, leaving good posterior condyles for the revision component, fixation will be compromised because bone has been lost from the posterior condyles as a result of the failed knee or the removal of components. That is the purpose of posterior femoral augments. They exist to fill in bone defects and consequently to stabilize the knee in flexion by enabling the surgeon to select an appropriately large femoral component.

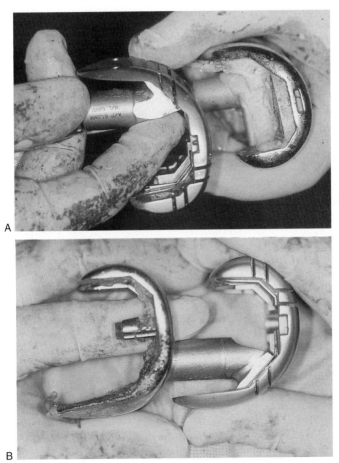

FIGURE 8.3. The femoral component is sized against the one removed. (A) If the knee was loose in flexion, a large femoral component is selected; or (B) if the original implant was sized correctly, a comparable revision femoral component is chosen.

Without them, we would be forced to use components that were too small.

In the presence of defective bone, due either to defects or soft quality, enhance fixation with medullary stems. These will influence the position of the femoral component and accordingly the stability of the knee in flexion. Stems can create problems. If large canal filling stems are selected, there will be little latitude for adjustment of the component position.[6] The component may be positioned in greater varus or valgus, flexion or extension or translated anteriorly or posteriorly, depending on the morphology of the femur. The position of smaller stems that are cemented in the canal (despite the undesirability of methacrylate in the canal) can be manipulated, anterior and posterior to affect the size of the flexion gap.

One situation that may arise when trying to determine the size of the femoral component is a gap mismatch. This important (and unusual) circumstance must be identified in any revision. Simply stated, a knee with an irreconcilable gap mismatch has a capacious flexion gap that, because of soft tissue failure, cannot be balanced to the likely dimensions of the extension gap with conventional releases or selection of the correct femoral component size. When the collateral ligaments, in particular the medial collateral, have stretched, it seems that we cannot find a femoral component large enough to stabilize the knee in flexion without an unacceptably thick polyethylene. The necessary femoral component may be so large that it no longer fits the medial to lateral dimensions of the bone. We have a knee that cannot be stabilized in flexion simply by recreating the anteroposterior dimensions of the femur.

The gap mismatch marks a decision point in the revision requiring a choice between accepting the laxity in flexion and protecting the patient with a constrained component or advancing the collateral ligament on the femur.[7] Our preference has been to avoid linked, constrained devices (hinges) in all cases, and to even reconstruct ligaments *and* use a nonlinked constrained device. With this decision noted, the femoral component size and position established and the tibial insert selected, the difficult work of the arthroplasty is complete.

(B) Seat the Femoral Component in External Rotation
The femoral component must be correctly rotated in the femoral canal. Internal rotation leads to patellar maltracking and a host of extensor mechanism problems. What landmarks exist for the correct rotation of the revision femur? There are two: the

epicondylar axis and the height of residual posterior condylar bone.

The epicondylar axis, an imaginary line joining the medial and lateral epicondyles (where the collateral ligaments attach to the femur) lies in variable amounts of external rotation. It defines the attachment of the collateral ligaments and accordingly their functional length. The residual posterior condylar bone, hidden in the back of the knee, is another reliable guide. Though not visible, it is palpable. With the knee flexed to 90 degrees, one can feel the residual bone above the posterior condyles, by running a finger up onto the posterior femoral cortex (Fig. 8.4). If there is much more bone left on the medial side as compared to the lateral side, we know that the failed femoral component had been implanted in internal rotation. The converse implies external rotation.

Again, do not be fooled by the residual bone and seat a revision femoral component in internal rotation. Defective bone should be reconstructed with augments. Use posterior augments preferentially on the lateral side to correct internal rotation.

(C) Reestablish the Joint Line

We have seen that stability in flexion is determined by the revision femoral component size and position. To fully stabilize the knee

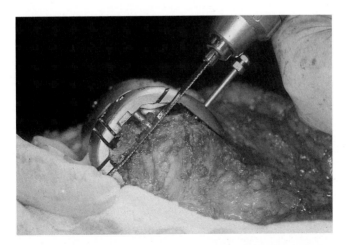

FIGURE 8.4. Rotational position of the femoral component can be determined by palpation of the posterior femoral condyles.

requires a polyethylene tibial insert so that the combined height of the posterior condyles of the femoral component and the tibial insert match the dimensions of the flexion gap. The point at which the femoral component meets the tibial polyethylene is the joint line. Where then does the patella lie? (Fig. 8.5)

The challenge for the surgeon is to match the prosthetic joint line height as closely as possible to the anatomic joint line. What is the best remaining landmark for approximating the anatomic joint line? The location of the inferior pole of the patella, when the knee is flexed to 90 degrees is an easily identified and reliable indicator of desired joint line. Ideally, the joint line should lie distal to the inferior pole of the patella. In choosing between two femoral component sizes, both of which stabilize the knee in flexion, but each of which requires different thicknesses of tibial polyethylene, select the combination that gives the best patellar height.

Step 3 Seat Femoral Component to Stabilize Knee in Extension (Figure 8.6)

This part is easy. The femoral component must be seated on the distal femur so that there is neither recurvatum nor a flexion contracture. If the trial components result in recurvatum, the femoral component may be seated more distally by using distal femoral augments. This will be the case in the majority of revisions in which

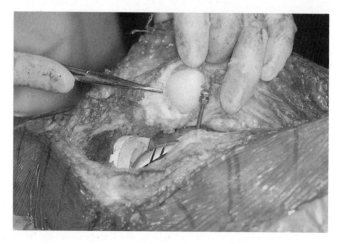

FIGURE 8.5. The point at which the femoral component meets the tibial articular surface is the joint line. The patella height is then noted.

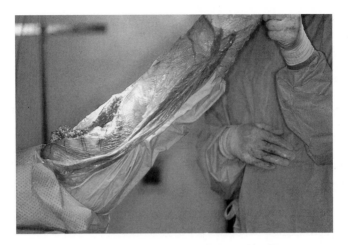

FIGURE 8.6. With the provisional components in place the knee is brought to full extension.

bone is missing as a result of failed primary. Selecting a thicker polyethylene tibial insert instead of a distal femoral augment will unbalance the stability that had been achieved in Step 2, in which the knee was stabilized in flexion.

Rarely, the surgeon may resect additional distal femur to stabilize the knee in extension. This may occur for the knee that had failed with a fixed flexion contracture, especially if the joint line had been *lowered* during the primary arthroplasty. When distal femoral resection is contemplated, check that it is not for the purpose of accommodating an inordinately thick tibial insert that is going to result in proximal joint line migration. This could be a gap mismatch.

DECISION POINT: SOFT TISSUE BALANCE IMPOSSIBLE?
In trying to stabilize the knee in extension it may become apparent that one or both of the collateral ligaments is deficient. A failed medial collateral, producing valgus instability, is the most disabling. When the medial collateral has suffered true plastic failure, it will not be possible to stabilize the knee by releasing the lateral side. Despite extensive lateral collateral releases, the medial ligament remains lax. All further releases simply lengthen the lateral side, and increasingly thick articular polyethylene creates a flexion contracture because the posterior structures are intact.[8] This is a decision point. The revision cannot be left without a functional

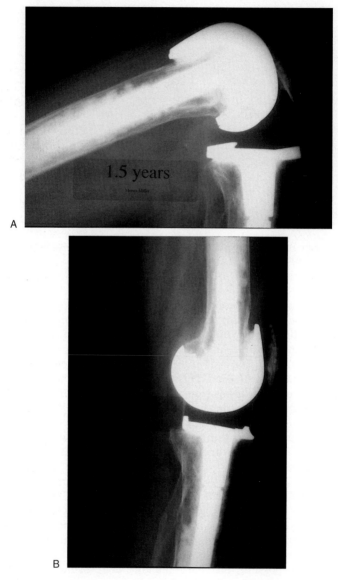

FIGURE 8.7. The revision arthroplasty should be stable in (A) flexion and (B) extension.

MCL and either a constrained implant or a ligament reconstruction (or both) will be required.

CONCLUSION

Having (1) reestablished the tibial platform, (2) stabilized the knee in flexion, and (3) stabilized the knee in extension, the revision arthroplasty is effectively complete. The trial components can be removed and the bone prepared for implantation of the permanent components. The three steps lend themselves to whatever implant is planned for the revision. Although posterior-stabilized implants generally provide a higher degree of stability for the revision, these steps can lead to a sound reconstruction when cruciate-retaining implants are selected. As has been indicated by the "decision points," circumstances arise when the pathology of the deformity dictates the best choice of implant.

The three steps to revision knee arthroplasty presented here provide the surgeon with an orderly approach based on sound surgical principles. Meticulous preoperative planning and adherence to the steps should allow the knee surgeon to overcome the daunting challenge of the revision knee arthroplasty (Fig. 8.7).

References

1. Vince KG. Revision Knee Arthroplasty Instructional Course Lectures of the AAOS. Mosby; 1992.
2. Vince K. Revision knee arthroplasty. In: Chapman, ed. *Operative Orthopedics*. Philadelphia: JB Lippincott; 1993:1981–2010.
3. Vince K. Planning revision total knee arthroplasty. *Seminars in Arthroplasty*; 1996.
4. Insall JN. Total knee replacement. In: Insall JN, ed. *Surgery of the Knee*. New York: Churchill Livingstone; 1984:587–696.
5. Vince KG, Insall JN. The total condylar knee arthroplasty. In: Laskin, ed. *Total Knee Arthroplasty*. New York: Springer Verlag; 1991.
6. Vince KG, Long W. Revision knee arthroplasty. The limits of press fit medullary fixation. *Clin Orthop*. August 1995; (317):172–177.
7. Vince K, Berkowitz R, Spitzer A. Ligament Reconstructions in Difficult Primary and Revision TKR. Accepted for presentation at the Annual Meeting of the Knee Society. San Francisco, California, February 1997.
8. Vince KG. Limb length discrepancy after revision total knee arthroplasty. *Techniques in Orthop*. 1988; 3:35–43.

Chapter 9
Classification of Bone Defects Femur and Tibia

Gerard A. Engh

An easy-to-use classification system that pinpoints the extent and location of bone damage helps surgeons plan efficiently for revision total knee surgery. Preoperative radiographs should be used to classify such bone defects into categories of comparable difficulty. Once surgeons determine the severity of bone loss, they can make well-informed decisions regarding the type of prosthesis to be used, the need for bone graft, and any special equipment the procedure may require.

When preparing for revision arthroplasty, the surgeon should anticipate the worst-case scenario. Revisions involving severe bone loss require skill, experience, and extra preparation, which may include practice on laboratory sawbone models. Appropriate classification followed by careful preparation and specialized treatment to repair bone damage should improve clinical results. When outcome studies are performed on these cases, the additional expense of modular revision systems would be warranted. In addition, a case mix based on bone defects can justify an implant comparison and validate clinical results.

HISTORICAL REVIEW OF BONE DEFECT CLASSIFICATION SCHEMES
Several attempts have been made to establish a classification of bone deficiencies for both primary and revision knee replacement surgery. In general, these schemes try to either categorize defects with similarities into a small number of defect types, or separate defects into a larger number of more specific groups.

Dorr's classification[1] is the most straightforward; defects are defined as either central or peripheral and cases are separated as primary or revision procedures. No attempt is made to define the size and location of the defect.

Insall[2] uses similar terminology in primary cases of central and peripheral bone defects. His classification is based on how to treat the defect: cement alone (stage 1); cement or augmentation plus a stemmed component (stage 2); or massive defects that require block augmentation and stem extension (stage 3).

In revision surgery, Insall's classification is primarily a visual description of bone defects that describes patterns of bone loss in both the femur and tibia. Femoral defects are categorized as symmetrical and asymmetrical distal loss, central and medial or lateral peg hole defects, distal ice cream cone, and asymmetrical ice cream cone deficiencies. Tibial deficiencies are categorized as proximal loss, asymmetrical loss, full slope, ice cream cone, asymmetrical ice cream cone, and contained defects.

Rand's classification is also based solely on the appearance of the defect at surgery. Rand's classification[3] differentiates three types of defects based on a combination of the depth of the defect and the percentage of the condyle involved. The most severe cavitary defect is further subdivided according to the integrity of the peripheral rim.

A comprehensive classification of bone deficiencies, which covers any and all defects of the femur, tibia, or patella, has been proposed by Bargar and Gross.[4] Four types of defects are defined for the femur and tibia and three types for the patella. Segmental, cavitary, and discontinuity defects can occur in any of the three locations, with intercalary defects as a fourth category for the tibia and femur. This scheme is similar to a classification system recommended by the Hip Society for defects adjacent to failed total hip implants. The large number of defects makes this classification cumbersome and somewhat impractical.

PREREQUISITES FOR A BONE DEFECT CLASSIFICATION

No bone defect classification has been accepted by orthopedic surgeons. Therefore, when the Anderson Orthopaedic Research Institute (AORI) bone defect classification was developed,[5] the goal was to make the system easy to understand and apply. The following criteria were the basis of the AORI classification:

1. The same terminology was employed for femoral and tibial defects because of the similarities in the metaphyseal segments of the femur and tibia.

2. The commonly used definitions in most classifications of bone defects, as central or peripheral, cortical or cancellous, contained or uncontained, were eliminated because of the absence of cortical bone in the metaphyseal segments of the distal femur and proximal tibia (Fig. 9.1).

3. Clear and precise definitions were established that minimize ambiguity when bone defects are categorized.

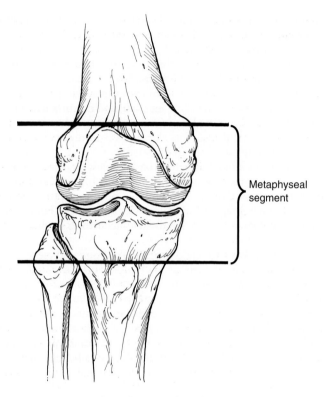

FIGURE 9.1. Metaphyseal region of the femur and tibia.

4. Aminimal number of defect types was established to permit clinical investigators to accumulate enough cases to allow meaningful statistical comparisons.

5. This classification was designed to allow retrospective categorization of cases through intraoperative information and postoperative radiographs.

X-RAY TECHNIQUE

It is important to have quality X-rays when classifying a bone defect. A true lateral view is essential to evaluate the location and extent of osteolysis that may be obscured by the prosthesis on an oblique radiograph. To obtain a "true" lateral view of the knee, the radiograph should be taken in 90 degrees of flexion, placing the entire leg, including the knee and ankle, flat on the radiograph table. If a true lateral view is not obtained, repeat radiographs should be performed after rotating the knee either internally or externally or moving the patient a few inches proximal or distal from the center of the beam.

AORI BONE DEFECT CLASSIFICATION

In this system, a defect is only classified when a component has been removed. If both the femoral and tibial components are removed, the femur and the tibia are each assigned a defect classification. Defects are classified from preoperative radiographs for anticipated bone deficiency and then the classification is either confirmed or changed intraoperatively. The femoral epicondyles, the posterior femoral condyles, and location of the patella relative to the joint line may be used as landmarks to differentiate complex femoral defects. The fibular head and the tibial tubercle should be used as landmarks for tibial defects that are difficult to classify.

Occasionally there is the need to classify a bone defect from postrevision radiographs. The metaphyseal segments of the femur and tibia have a distinct profile (Fig. 9.1). The main criterion to look for is a reduction in this profile and the dimensions of the metaphyseal segments of the femoral condyles and/or the tibial plateaus. The distance from the epicondyle to the end of the femur varies according to an individual's bone structure and size, but this distance is proportional to all other dimensions of the bone. A bone defect, however, alters this relationship. For example, a shortened distance from the epicondyle and metaphyseal flare to the end of the femoral component will be visible if a distal bone defect has not been repaired with a bone graft or an augment to restore a normal joint line. If the bone defects were reconstructed with cement, augments, or grafts and the joint line restored, this will be evident on postrevision radiographs and also in the patient's operative note. On the radiograph, the metaphyseal bone segment should appear as a shortened segment, with an augmented component or bone graft filling the deficient area.

Therefore, the following definitions are the foundation of this classification:

Type 1 Defect (INTACT metaphyseal bone): Minor bone defects that do not compromise the stability of the component.
Type 2 Defect (DAMAGED metaphyseal bone): Loss of cancellous bone that necessitates an area of cement fill, augments, or bone graft to restore a reasonable joint line level. Type 2 bone defects can occur in one-femoral condyle or tibial plateau (2A), or in both condyles or plateaus (2B).

Type 3 Defect (DEFICIENT metaphyseal segment): Bone loss
that compromises a major portion of either condyle or plateau.
These defects are occasionally associated with collateral or
patellar ligament detachment and usually require bone grafts
or custom implants.

In any classification scheme, some cases will fall on the bor-
derline. To classify these cases, it is necessary to evaluate the postoperative radiographs and the surgical treatment mode. For
example, if a primary component was used, no bone defect was
addressed in the operative note, and the postoperative radiographs
demonstrate joint line restoration, an F3/T3 defect would not apply.
If a structural bone graft, major cement fill, or a hinged component with condylar resection was used in the revision, we would
conclude that the patient had a significant F2/T2 or F3/T3 bone
defect.

Bone defects also occur in the patella but are not classified in
the AORI bone defect classification. Patellar defects were excluded
because they do not affect management decisions with revision
surgery. In these cases, bone grafting is not an option and revision
components to address such defects are not available, except for
the biconvex patellar design of the Genesis Knee (Smith & Nephew,
Memphis, TN). In most instances patellar bone defects are
managed simply by not resurfacing the damaged patellar bone.

FEMORAL BONE DEFECT

F1 Defects (Figure 9.2)
The preoperative radiographs of the Type 1 femur demonstrate a
correctly aligned component with no evidence of femoral osteolysis. They also show no significant component migration, and a
normal joint line level is indicated by patellar height and epicondyle to implant distance. On an anteroposterior radiograph, the
quality of bone appears to be strong enough in the metaphyseal
segment of the femur to support a component without a stem. The
dimensions of the posterior femoral condyles are full, allowing substitution of an implant of the same size with normal condylar
dimensions. An augmented component or a modular wedge is not
needed to restore joint line level. Minor surface irregularities from
cement plugs are managed with particulate bone graft or cement.
Table 9.1 summarizes the features and treatment modalities of an
F1 defect.

The postoperative radiographs of a Type 1 femur show a relatively normal joint line level with the patella about 1 cm proximal

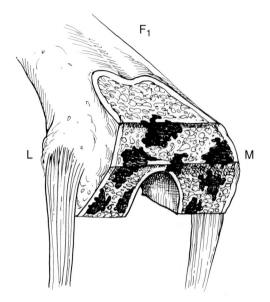

FIGURE 9.2. F1 Defect.

to the tibial plateau. The femoral condyles appear full on the anteroposterior radiograph; the posterior condylar offset created by preserving the posterior condylar bone is evident on the lateral radiograph. The proximal tip of the component's posterior condyle should match the proximal end of the patient's posterior femoral condyle.

F2 Defects

The F2 femoral bone defect is characterized by osteolysis or significant proximal migration of the femoral component. Radiographs may reveal subsidence of the implant with a circumferential radiolucency. Also, the loss of distance from the epicondyles to the end of the implant will be apparent on the anteroposterior radiograph. Femoral osteolysis should not extend above the epicondyles.

In some F2 defects, the normal relationship of the femoral component to the shaft of the femur (6 degrees valgus) is altered. The implant subsides with angular migration into an incorrect varus or valgus posture relative to the anatomic axis of the femur. The F2A defect often demonstrates an increased varus or valgus orientation of the femoral component (from the normal 6 degrees). In an F2A

TABLE 9.1. Guideline for classifying defects

Defect type	Identifying features	Treatment
F1/T1	no component subsidence or osteolysis; no cancellous defects in the peripheral rim; cancellous bone that will support an implant; defects can be filled by small amounts of particulate bone graft or cement; a normal joint line is present	no augments (>4 mm), structural grafts, or cement fill (>1 cm);
		no stemmed components necessary
	femur—full condylar profile	
	tibia—component above the fibular head and a full metaphyseal segment	
F2/T2	cancellous bone inadequate to support the implant; cancellous defects may require bone grafts; the component used requires augmentation to restore the joint line; osteolysis may be more extensive than radiographs indicate	joint line restored with an augmented component (>4 mm), particulate autograft or allograft, or cement fill (>1 cm);
	femur—reduced condylar profile	stemmed components should be used
	tibia—component is at or below the tip of the fibular head and the tibial flare is reduced	
F3/T3	marked component migration; knee instability; deficient metaphyseal segment	structural graft, augment or cement, or a hinged component used to reconstruct the condyle or plateau;
	femur—loss of collateral ligament attachments from one or both condyles; severe condylar bone loss from osteolysis or a comminuted supracondylar fracture	stemmed components required

defect, bone of the uninvolved condyle is present at a normal joint line level. See Table 9.1 for a summary of bone defects.

F2A Defects: One Condyle (Figure 9.3)

A Type 2A femur can involve either condyle. The cancellous bone of the involved condyle may have been damaged by osteolysis or iatrogenically if an incorrect angular resection of the distal femur was made at the time of the primary arthroplasty. The bone of the opposite femoral condyle is relatively intact near a normal joint line level.

The radiographic criterion for a Type 2A femur is the presence of unilateral elevation of the joint line with adequate bone in the opposite condyle for component fixation. The presence of minor bone defects in the opposite condyle does not alter the classification of a Type 2A defect as long as the opposite condyle maintains a relatively normal joint line level.

Reconstruction of an F2A defect with a primary implant is rarely indicated. In most instances, the damaged condyle should be repaired with a modular augment to restore a normal joint line. In some circumstances, an F2A defect should be treated with

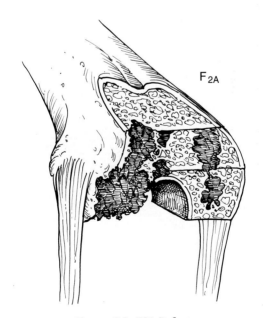

FIGURE 9.3. F2A Defect.

incomplete joint line restoration. This may be necessary to correct a large preoperative flexion contracture. An F2A defect is converted to an F2B defect when the opposite condyle is resected at a more proximal level. When the joint line is elevated, a smaller femoral component is needed to restore flexion-extension balance.

Postoperative radiographs of a correctly reconstructed F2A defect should show the augmented or repaired condyle. The antero-posterior radiograph may demonstrate the more proximal resection level of the condyle. However, an augment is not always visible on the lateral radiograph if it is hidden by the box of a posterior-stabilized or more constrained implant.

F2B Defect: Both Condyles (Figure 9.4)
The defect in a Type 2B femur is identical to the Type 2A defect except that it involves both femoral condyles. The damaged meta-physeal bone requires reconstruction of both condyles with bone, cement, or augments to restore an acceptable joint line level. Cases of multiple revisions and failure of stemmed femoral components often create Type 2B defects.

On the anteroposterior radiograph of a subsided femoral component, the distance from the distal end of the component to the

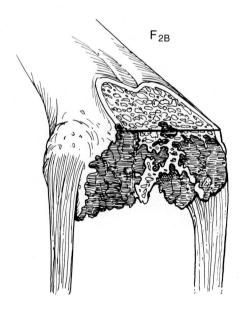

FIGURE 9.4. F2B Defect.

epicondyles appears to have decreased. If the epicondyles are flared by component migration, the defect is extensive and indicative of an F3 defect. On an anteroposterior radiograph, osteolysis may be visible in the bone between the component and the metaphyseal edge of the bone. Also, patella baja may be present on the lateral radiograph. With proximal migration of the prosthetic joint line, the posterior condyle of the component may have migrated to a position above the patient's remaining posterior femoral condyle. Extensive cement fill proximal to a femoral component usually results in an F2B classification.

It is often necessary to augment both femoral condyles distally and posteriorly by using modular wedges to restore joint line level. Cement fill, sometimes reinforced with cancellous bone screws at the base of the defect, may be used to replace lost bone when the interface is not good for cement bonding. An F2B defect should always be revised with a stemmed component.

Some F2B defects require joint line elevation to restore adequate knee motion. This is true in a stiff knee with a flexion contracture greater than 20 degrees. If a release of the contracted posterior capsule proves inadequate, joint line elevation without augmentation may be needed to correct the patient's flexion contracture. A stemmed revision component should be used.

The postoperative radiographs of an F2B defect demonstrate either joint line elevation without repair of a major bone defect, or a joint line that has been restored with augments, bone graft, or a thick mantle of cement beneath the component. The metaphyseal segment of bone will appear shortened and replaced by the increased thickness of the femoral component. Bone grafts may be difficult to see if the graft is in close apposition to host bone and if the host bone has been sufficiently reamed to a cancellous bed. The patella may be at or below the top of the tibial component, thereby indicating joint line elevation.

F3 Defect (Figure 9.5)
Type 3 femoral defects have extensive structural bone loss, involving a major portion of one or both femoral condyles. See Table 9.1 for identifying features of F3 defects.

The preoperative radiographs of F3 defects demonstrate osteolysis and/or severe component migration to the level of the epicondyles. When the femur migrates, the epicondyles flare away from the component. Although the severity of osteolysis is not always apparent on radiographs, the surgeon should assume that osteolysis is present and may be far more severe than anticipated. Osteolysis usually appears as a defect in the cancellous bone adja-

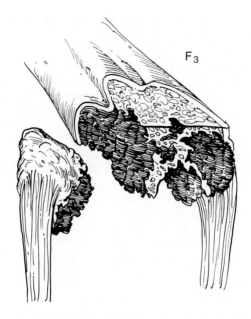

FIGURE 9.5. F3 Defect.

cent to the implant. The most common locations are at the margins
of the femoral component, and usually appear with a sclerotic and
scalloped border. Lytic lesions of osteolysis frequently begin in
areas where the femoral component is not bonded to underlying
host bone.[6] Although many osteolytic defects demonstrate a
sclerotic border, the most aggressive lesions may not have this
radiographic feature.

Failure of a hinged, custom, or revision component often
results in an F3 defect. These components devices often have stems
that migrate in the axis of the femur. A significant amount of bone
is lost or sacrificed when these devices are implanted. In these
cases, the expanded metaphyseal segment of the femur is
shortened.

The surgical reconstruction of an F3 defect is a salvage type
procedure requiring a major replacement of metaphyseal bone
with either a structural allograft or a custom femoral component.
The extensive bone loss may involve one or both condyles. A varus-
valgus constrained implant, or preservation and reattachment of
one or both collateral ligaments, may be necessary. In this case,
a canal-filling stem is required. Rotational stability of the femoral

component may require fully cementing the stem or step cutting the allograft and host bone.

The postoperative radiographs of Type 3 femurs demonstrate the reconstruction of a segment of the distal femoral metaphysis and in some instances, diaphysis. Hinged devices are classified as F3 defects because they replace the metaphyseal segment and are recognized by the linkage joining the two components. Demarcation of the allograft from adjacent host bone is often evident because of the differing density of bone and the slower bridging and remodeling that occur if the graft involves the diaphyseal region. The ideal reconstruction of an F3 defect includes restoring the normal joint line using a polyethylene insert of normal thickness.

TIBIAL BONE DEFECT

The same principles used in classifying femoral defects apply to tibial bone deficiencies. Component loosening is more common in tibial implants. Frequently, the tibial prosthesis subsides into varus, creating a bone defect in the medial tibial plateau. Canal-filling stems should be used in cases of large bone defects and whenever increased prosthetic constraint is required for knee stability.

T1 Defect (Figure 9.6)

The Type 1 tibia has the same identifying features as the F1 femoral defect (see Table 9.1). Preoperative radiographs reveal a correctly aligned tibial component without significant implant subsidence or tibial osteolysis. There is a full flare to the proximal tibia and the bone is present above the patellar ligament and the fibular head. A standard tibial component is recommended for T1 defects because there is adequate cancellous host bone.

Postoperative radiographs confirm that bone has been preserved above the fibular head and that the fullness and contour of the tibial metaphysis have been maintained. Usually a standard component was used with a combined polyethylene and metal thickness of less than 20mm.

T2 Defect

The T2 defect is often caused by component loosening and secondary subsidence of the tibia, commonly into a varus orientation. A circumferential radiolucency develops between the cement and bone as the component subsides. The distance between the top of the fibula and the component is diminished. The lateral radiograph is useful in measuring this distance. Osteolysis may present as cav-

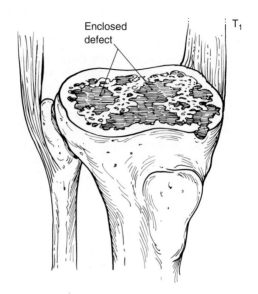

FIGURE 9.6. T1 Defect.

itary defects beneath the component. See Table 9.1 for a summary of tibial defects.

T2A Defect: One Plateau (Figure 9.7)

The Type 2A defect is usually the result of tibial component loosening and subsiding into varus. The tibia rarely subsides into a valgus orientation, even in knees with valgus alignment. On preoperative radiographs, a widening radiolucency is frequently seen beneath the tibial component. Bone in the opposite tibial plateau is present at a relatively normal joint line level. T2A defects can also occur with aseptic loosening of a unicondylar tibial component.

The surgical management of a T2A defect includes the use of a stemmed implant along with a small bulk autograft, allograft, or a wedged tibial component. The augment can be a horizontal step wedge, a half wedge, or a whole wedge. It is important to avoid converting a T2A defect into a T2B defect by resecting the tibial plateau at a more distal level. When a T2B defect is created iatrogenically, a thicker tibial component is required.

T2B Defect: Both Plateaus (Figure 9.8)

The Type 2B defect (Fig. 9.8) involves both plateaus. Radiographs of T2B defects demonstrate damage to the metaphyseal segment of

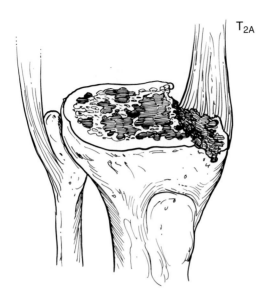

FIGURE 9.7. T2A Defect.

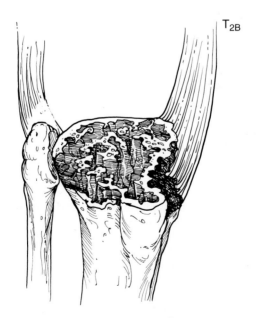

FIGURE 9.8. T2B Defect.

the tibia by either component subsidence, osteolysis, or both. The damage may extend to the level of the fibular head, but should not include extensive destruction of bone below this level. The metaphyseal flare of the tibia should be reduced but still present. Osteolytic lesions should have a well-defined border with some cancellous bone present for cement interdigitation at the time of the reconstruction.

The surgical management of a T2B defect usually includes the use of a long-stemmed tibial component and reconstruction of the tibial plateaus by bone graft, augments, or an extra thick tibial component. A wedgeshaped component is appropriate for the T2B defect if the bone loss is significant in both plateaus, but greater in one plateau. A canal-filling stem is preferable, particularly if a structural bone graft has been used.

Occasionally, cement fill is used for T2B defect reconstructions. Reinforcement with cancellous screws may provide a stronger construct than cement alone. The most difficult but perhaps the most important aspect of Type 2 and Type 3 tibial reconstructions is achieving cement interdigitation with the graft. An advantage to using allograft bone is recreating a cancellous bone bed for cement interdigitation with host bone. Union of an allograft to host bone is not a problem.[7] In fact, the durability of major structural allografts in revision knee surgery appears to be satisfactory.

Postoperative radiographs of T2B repairs reveal a tibial component augment, cement fill, or allograft to restore joint line level. The augment may be an extra thick tibial baseplate, a step wedge, or an angular wedge beneath the component. There may be a bone graft in addition to the augment. If the defect has not been repaired to restore joint line level, the tibial baseplate is at or below the level of the fibular head. In some instances, the tibial baseplate may be close to the fibular head, with extensive cement penetration below the level of the fibular head.

T3 Defect (Figure 9.9)

The Type 3 tibial defect usually results from severe tibial component instability caused by aseptic loosening and implant migration. Osteolysis or an underlying bone fracture may contribute to the development of T3 defects. The T3 tibial defect has extensively damaged cancellous bone of the proximal tibia. The fibular head may be retained, leaving it higher than the proximal tibia. A canal-filling stem must be used to support the component. In severe cases, the metaphyseal flare of the tibia is completely absent. This situation requires a major structural allograft to repair the proximal tibial segment for joint line restoration and component fixation.

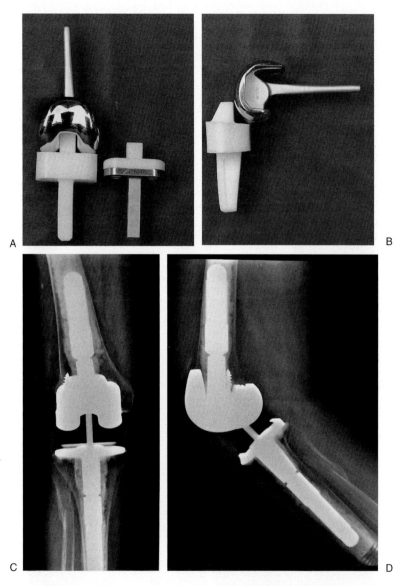

FIGURE 10.1. (A) Anteroposterior and (B) lateral photograph and (C) anteroposterior and (D) lateral radiograph of total condylar III prosthesis.

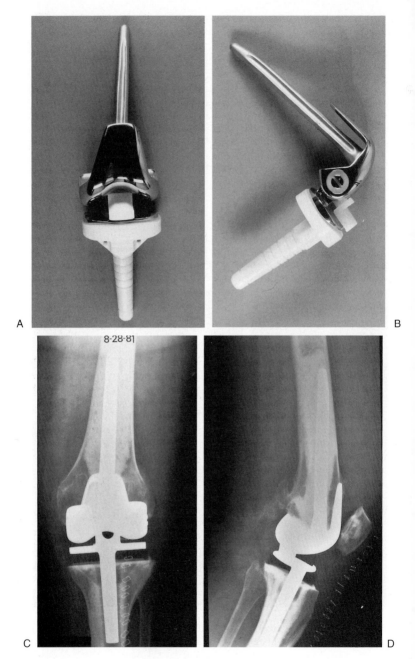

FIGURE 10.2. (A) Anteroposterior and (B) lateral photograph and (C) anteroposterior and (D) lateral radiograph of kinematic rotating hinge prosthesis.

FIGURE 10.3. (A) Anteroposterior and (B) lateral photograph of Noiles rotating hinge prosthesis.

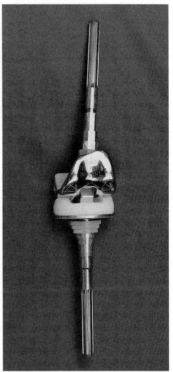

A

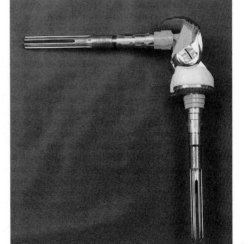

B

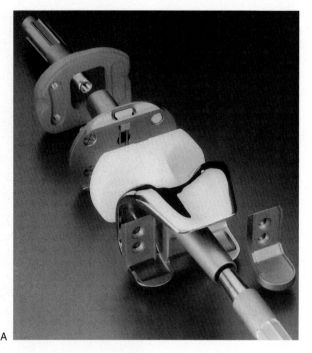

A

FIGURE 10.4. (A) Photograph, (B) anteroposterior and (C) lateral radiograph of constrained condylar total knee prosthesis.

be added to the undersurface of the tibia for similar reasons (Figs. 10.4A–C).

The type of intra-articular constraint desired may also be varied with modular total knee systems depending upon the clinical setting. A posterior-stabilized or cruciate-retaining tibial polyethylene implant may be used, or, in situations in which instability is greater, a more constrained tibial polyethylene component may be used that provides a thick intercondylar peg similar to the total condylar III design.

INDICATIONS

Constrained total knee prostheses have been selected for a wide variety of reasons. The most common reasons for use of a constrained prosthesis are ligamentous instability,[4,6,7,10,11,13,15–17,20] bone

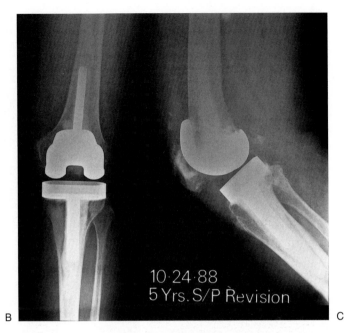

B   C

FIGURE 10.4. *Continued.*

loss,[4,7,11,15] deformity,[6,10,16] revision of a prior failed TKA,[6,10,13,16] septic or aseptic loosening,[11,17,20] or supracondylar femur fracture[15,20] (Figs. 10.5A–E). Additional indications for use of a constrained prosthesis are cases of unstable revision in which a resurfacing arthroplasty will not suffice,[10] anticipated heavy use of the knee,[6] implant malposition,[15] inadvertent transection of the medial collateral ligament during standard total knee arthroplasty,[13] extreme imbalance in the flexion-extension gaps,[20] recurrent dislocation of previous posterior-stabilized constrained knee arthroplasty,[20] and exposure obtained by the so-called "femoral peel."[8,20] The authors limit the use of constrained designs to knees with a deficient collateral ligament, supracondylar femur fracture with extensive bone loss in an elderly patient, or cases with large soft tissue imbalance after appropriate ligament releases.

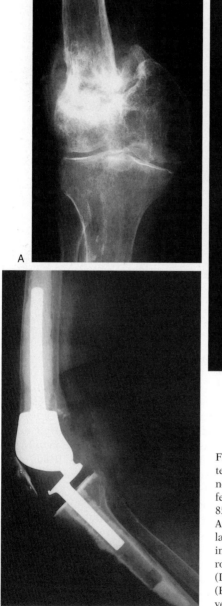

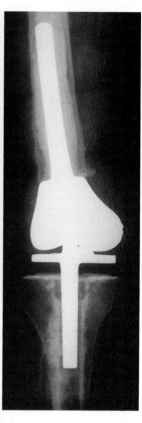

FIGURE 10.5. (A) Anteroposterior radiograph of nonunion of supracondylar femur fracture in an 85-year-old woman. (B) Anteroposterior and (C) lateral radiographs following custom kinematic rotating hinge total knee. (D) Anteroposterior and (E) lateral radiographs at 5 years following revision.

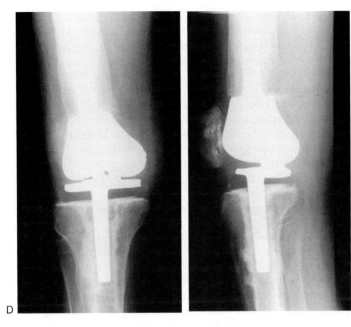

D   E

FIGURE 10.5. *Continued.*

RESULTS

The results of revision TKA using constrained devices are variable and affected by prosthesis design, surgical technique, and length of follow-up. Most studies have demonstrated inferior results to primary knee replacement procedures. It is important, however, to view these results in light of the evolving technical aspects of revision total knee replacement and the improvements in implants used for these revision procedures.

Hinge Prostheses for Revision

The largest and most recent series for revision TKA using constrained prosthesis, to date, is reported by Lombardi.[20] Using the Hospital for Special Surgery rating system, they studied 113 rotating hinge revision TKAs. The mean follow-up was 6 years. Eighteen knees (16%) were rated excellent, 58 knees (51%) were rated good, 26 knees (23%) were rated fair, and 11 knees (10%) were rated poor.

Rand and associates[7] reported the results of 23 kinematic rotating hinge total knee arthroplasties used for revision at the Mayo Clinic. Using the Hospital for Special Surgery scoring system, at a mean of 50 months, of the revision knees 9 (39%) were rated excellent, 7 (30%) good, 3 (13%) fair, 2 (9%) poor, and 2 were unavailable for follow-up.

Shaw and colleagues[11] reported the results of revision using the kinematic rotating hinge prosthesis using the Brigham and Women's Hospital and Harvard Medical School knee rating system. Mean follow-up was 50 months; 22% had excellent results, 40% had good results, 13% had fair results, and more than 10% had poor results. Shindell and associates reported on 18 Noiles hinged prostheses of which 4 were revisions.[6] All 4 revisions failed at a mean of 31 months. Femoral component subsidence occurred in 17 of 18 knees.

Total Condylar III Prostheses for Revision

Lombardi,[20] using the Hospital for Special Surgery rating system, reported 66 revision TKAs using a posterior-stabilized constrained prosthesis. The posterior-stabilized constrained prosthesis had a mean follow-up of 14 months; 19 knees (30%) were rated excellent, 36 knees (53%) were rated good, 6 knees (9%) were rated fair, and 5 knees (8%) were rated poor.

Donaldson and colleagues[10] studied 31 knees in 25 patients using the total condylar III knee prosthesis. There were 17 primary arthroplasties and 14 revisions with an average follow-up period of 3.8 years. Using the Hospital for Special Surgery knee-rating score for the revision arthroplasties, 2 (14%) were rated as excellent, 5 (36%) were rated as good, 1 (7%) was rated as fair, and 1 (7%) was rated as poor. There were 5 (36%) failures.

Kavolus and associates[13] studied the total condylar III knee prosthesis in elderly patients. Sixteen knee arthroplasties were performed in 14 patients with 11 of the 16 being revisions. Mean follow-up was 4.5 years. In this age group, 15 of 16 implants had a good or excellent Hospital for Special Surgery knee score.

Rand and colleagues[15] reported revision TKA using the total condylar III prosthesis in 21 knees in 19 patients. At 4-year follow-up using the Hospital for Special Surgery knee score, 25% were excellent, 25% were good, 25% were fair, and 25% were poor. The results were not influenced by the number of prior revisions or the prior prosthesis type.

Rosenberg and associates[17] also reported the clinical results of total knee revision using the total condylar III prosthesis. At mean follow-up of 45 months, 11 patients (30%) were graded excellent, 14 patients (39%) good, 6 (17%) fair, 4 (11%) poor, and there was one failure.

Hohl reported the results of the total condylar III prosthesis in complex knee reconstruction at a mean of 6.1 years for 29 revised TKAs.[16] Using the Knee Society scoring system, 71% of the patients had good or excellent results.

Kim reported the results of fourteen hinge prostheses that were revised to a total condylar III design.[8] The patients were followed for 4 years. The Hospital for Special Surgery Knee Score improved from 58 to 81.

The results of Lombardi and Hohl are similar to those reported by Rand, Donaldson, Shaw, Kavolus, and Rosenberg, which demonstrate 50 to 92% of the patients with good or excellent results following revision TKA using constrained devices (Table 10.1).

COMPLICATIONS

Stuart and associates[19] discussed various reasons for reoperation after knee revision surgery that included implant loosening, sepsis, extensor mechanism problems, fractures of bone or prosthetic components, wear debris, and limited range of motion. The most common complications following revision TKA using constrained devices involve problems with the patella. Walker[4] in a series of 22 knees (21 revisions) noted one patellar subluxation and one patellar dislocation. Rand[7] in a series of 38 knees (23 revisions) noted patellar instability in 9, patellar implant loosening in 2, patellar fractures in 2, and patellar tendon ruptures in 2 knees. Shaw[11] noted in a series of 38 knees (18 revisions) that 36% of the revisions had perioperative patellar subluxation. Many other authors have elucidated problems with the extensor mechanism following revision TKA using constrained prostheses.[10,13–17,20]

Inglis and colleagues[14] noted that a major complication and cause of failure of revision total knee arthroplasty was fracture of the femur at the level of the tip of the intramedullary stem. This was due to the close proximity of the tip to the lateral cortex. This complication occurred in 38% of the first revisions and in 31% of the second revisions, comprising more than half the failures.

TABLE 10.1. Results of revision total knee arthroplasty using constrained devices

Author	Number	Follow-Up	Excellent	Good	Fair	Poor	Failures
Rand et al.[7]*	38 Knees (21 revised)	4.2 years	9 (43%)	7 (33%)	3 (14%)	2 (9%)	0
Donaldson et al.[10]*	31 Knees (14 revised)	3.8 years	2 (14%)	5 (36%)	1 (7%)	1 (7%)	5 (36%)
Kavolus et al.[13]*	16 Knees (11 revised)	4.2 years	5 (45%)	5 (45%)	1 (9%)	0	0
Rand et al.[15]*	21 Knees	4.0 years	5 (24%)	5 (24%)	5 (24%)	4 (19%)	1 (5%)
Hohl et al.[16]**	35 Knees (29 revised)	6.1 years	18 (51%)	7 (20%)	2 (6%)	5 (14%)	3 (9%)
Rosenberg et al.[17]**	36 Knees	3.75 years	11 (30%)	14 (39%)	6 (17%)	4 (11%)	1 (3%)
Lombardi et al.[20]*	113 Knees	2.1 years	18 (16%)	58 (51%)	26 (23%)	11 (10%)	0

(*) Hospital for Special Surgery Score
(**) Knee Society Score

Donaldson and associates[10] noted failures included three prostheses removed for deep infections. Additional failures included aseptic loosening in two knees. Hohl and colleagues[16] noted three failures (8.6%); two failures were from infection and one from implant loosening.

Rosenberg and associates[17] noted four hemarthroses, four patients with chronic and symptomatic patellar subluxation, one superficial wound infection, one symptomatic deep vein thrombosis, one pulmonary embolism, one cerebrovascular accident, and one late neuroma. Two knee manipulations were required to gain flexion, one of which suffered a femoral fracture at manipulation that healed after cast brace treatment. One metal-backed patella was revised for excessive wear.

Rand[16] noted that complications consisted of two atraumatic patellar fractures, one patellar tendon rupture, one transient skin ischemia, one superficial infection, one deep infection, and one nonunion of a preexisting supracondylar femur fracture. Two of the extensor mechanism complications adversely affected the results with two poor and only one good knee score. The one transient skin ischemia resolved with cessation of knee motion, and the patient had an excellent knee score. The one deep infection required an above-knee amputation for control of sepsis. The patient who had revision using a cemented long-stem femoral component for a preexisting supracondylar femur fracture developed nonunion at the fracture site and had a poor knee score.

Other complications following revision TKA using constrained devices include breakage, loosening, superficial infection, deep infections, arthrofibrosis, femur and/or tibial shaft fractures, peroneal nerve palsies, shortening, nonunion, and screw disengagements (Table 10.2).

CONCLUSIONS

The need of constraint is relatively infrequent in primary versus revision total knee arthroplasty. Indications include deficient collateral ligaments, inadequate soft tissue balancing that cannot be salvaged, and marked metaphyseal bone loss (i.e, supracondylar femur or proximal tibia). The results of revision arthroplasty in this difficult group of patients will be satisfactory in 50% with a complication rate of 30 to 50%. Our preference is to use the least amount of constraint for revision.

TABLE 10.2. Complications of revision total knee arthroplasty using constrained devices

Author	Number	Patellar	Tibial	Femoral	Loosening	Sup. Infection
Walker et al.[4]	21 revisions	1 subluxation; 1 dislocation	1 avulsion of tubercle; 1 shaft perforation	2 shaft perforations		
Rand et al.[7]	23 revisions	9 instabilities 2 loosening; 2 tendon rupture; 2 fracture		2 fractures	3 with aseptic leading to revision (2/3)	6
Donaldson et al.[10]	14 revisions	1 fracture			2 with aseptic loosening	
Shaw et al.[11]	18 revisions	36% revisions with subluxation	1 fracture			3
Kavolus et al.[13] Inglis et al.[14] Rand[15]	11 revisions 40 revisions 21 Knees	2 dislocations 1 ligament rupture 2 fractures; 1 tendon rupture	1 fracture 2 fractures	14 fractures		1
Hohl et al.[16] Rosenberg et al.[17]	29 revisions 36 Knees	1 subluxation 4 subluxations; 1 metal backed revised for excessive wear		1 fracture	2 aseptic loosening	1
Lombardi et al.[20]	113 Knees	1 subluxation; 2 fractures			6 femoral component loosening secondary to allograft failure	2

Deep Infection	Breakage	Arthrofibrosis	Wound	Bleeding	Nerve Palsies	Other
8	8					
8		1 knee manipulation	5 wound complications	2 intra-articular bleeding	1 peroneal nerve palsy	1 shortening > 60mm; 1 removal of cement debris
1			1 transient skin ischemia			1 non-union of a pre-existing supracondylar fracture
2		3 knee manipulations	1 wound slough; 1 decubitus ulcer		2 peroneal nerve palsies	1 tibial post dislocation
1		2 knee manipulations		4 hematomas		1 DVT; 1 PE; 1 late neuroma
4		5 knee manipulations				2 femoral-tibial dislocations; 2 screw disengagements

References

1. Levens AS, Berkeley CE, Inman VT, and Blosser JA. Transverse rotation of the segments of the lower extremity in locomotion. *J Bone Joint Surg.* 1948; 30A:859–872.

2. Nogi J, Caldwell JW, Kavzlanich JJ, Thompson RC Jr. Load testing of geometric and polycentric total knee replacement. *Clin Orthop.* 1976; 114:235–242.

3. Accardo NJ, Noiles DG, Pena R, Accardo NJ Jr. Noiles total knee replacement procedure. *Orthopedics.* 1979; 2:37–45.

4. Walker PS, Emerson R, Potter T, Scott R, Thomas WH, Turner RH. The kinematic rotating hinge: biomechanics and clinical application. *Orthop Clin of North Am.* 1982; 13(1):187–199.

5. Rand JA, Peterson LFA, Bryan RS, Ilstrup DM. Revision total knee arthroplasty. Instructional Course Lectures XXXV: 1986:305–318.

6. Shindell R, Neumann R, Connolly JF, Jardon OM. Evaluation of the Noiles hinged knee prosthesis. *J Bone Joint Surg.* 1986; 68A(4):579–585.

7. Rand JA, Chao YS, Stauffer RN. Kinematic rotating-hinge total knee arthroplasty. J Bone Joint Surg. 1987; 69A(4):489–497.

8. Kim YH. Salvage of failed hinge knee arthroplasty with a total condylar III type prosthesis. *Clin Orthop.* 1987; 221:272–277.

9. Sculco TP. Total condylar III prosthesis in ligament instability. *Orthop Clin of North Am.* 1989; 20(2):221–226.

10. Donaldson WF, Sculco TP, Insall JN, Ranawat CS. Total condylar III knee prosthesis—long-term follow-up study. *Clin Orthop.* 1988; 226:21–28.

11. Shaw JA, Balcom W, Greer RB. Total knee arthroplasty using the kinematic rotating hinge prosthesis. *Orthopedics.* 1989; 12(5):647–654.

12. Goldberg VM, ed. *Controversies of Total Knee Arthroplasty.* New York: Raven Press, 1991.

13. Kavolus CH, Faris PM, Ritter MA, Keating EM. The total condylar III knee prosthesis in elderly patients. *J of Arthroplasty.* 1991; 6(1):39–43.

14. Inglis AE, Walker PS. Revision of failed knee replacements using fixed-axis hinges. *J Bone Joint Surg.* 1991; 73B(5):757–761.

15. Rand JA. Revision total knee arthroplasty using the total condylar III prosthesis. *J of Arthroplasty.* 1991; 6(3):279–284.

16. Hohl WM, Crawfurd E, Zelicof SB, Ewald FC. The total condylar III prosthesis in complex knee reconstruction. *Clin Orthop.* 1991; 273:91–97.

17. Rosenberg AG, Verner JJ, Galante JO. Clinical results of total knee revision using the total condylar III prosthesis. *Clin Orthop.* 1991; 273:83–90.

18. Morgan CL, Rand JA. Results of total knee arthroplasty using older constrained implant designs. In: Rand JA, ed. Total *Knee Arthroplasty.* New York: Raven Press; 1993:177–191.

19. Stuart MJ, Larson JE, Morrey F. Reoperation after condylar revision total knee arthroplasty. *Clin Orthop.* 1993; 286:168–173.
20. Lombardi AV Jr, Mallory TH, Eberle RW, Adams JB. Results of revision total knee arthroplasty using constrained prostheses. *Seminars in Arthroplasty*, in press, 1996.

Chapter 11
Two-Stage Reimplantation for Infection

Giles R. Scuderi and Henry D. Clarke

Two-stage reimplantation of infected total knee arthroplasty has become the treatment of choice for most patients.[1,2,3,4] The treatment protocol is divided into three phases: (1) removal of the prosthesis and all cement with debridement of the soft tissues and bone; (2) six weeks of parental antibiotics; and (3) implantation of a new total knee prosthesis. To have adequate bone stock for the later reimplantation, care should be taken at the time of component removal care. While all attempts to perform a thorough debridement and cement removal are undertaken, overzealous debridement can lead to significant bone loss, complicating the reimplantation.

Following the removal of the infected components, cement spacers are placed between the femoral–tibial and patellofemoral articulations. The use of antibioticimpregnated cement beads or spacer blocks allows local delivery of high concentrations of antibiotics. While the larger surface area of multiple beads theoretically provides greater allusion of local antibiotics than from a single spacer block, no definite clinical advantage has been proven. However, the spacer block has definite mechanical advantages over the beads. Spacer blocks facilitate ambulation prior to the reimplantation and also allow easier exposure at the time of the later surgery.[5] In most cases a spacer block is fashioned using two to three 40 g batches of polymethylmethacrylate cement mixed with high doses of antibiotics. We typically use 2.4 g of tobramycin and 1 g of vancomycin per pack of cement. When mixing the antibiotics, the lumps in the crystalline vancomycin should not be crushed. Once the cement has reached a doughy consistency it is placed into the femoral tibial space during the final stages of polymerization. Longitudinal distraction is applied to the extremity in an effort to prevent cement interdigitation with the bone; this enables easy removal at the time of reimplantation. If large spacers are used, the heat produced by the exothermic reaction can be significant. Irrigation should be used to cool the cement block, preventing damage to the neurovascular structures that lie only millimeters from the posterior capsule. The cement spacer can be fashioned with short pegs or stems to help provide stability. Extending the spacer anteriorly over the distal femur and into the patellofemoral joint also helps with stability and maintains a plane between the patella and femur. The block should be suitably large to sit on cortical bone and provide stability in extension. If the block is too small and has contact predominantly with cancellous bone or is insufficient to maintain stability, further bone erosion can occur. If the intramedullary canal is opened to remove stemmed components, antibiotic-impregnated cement rods can be placed inside the canals. Use of a cement spacer usually provides enough stability to the knee to allow the patient to walk for short distances in a knee immobilizer, brace, or cast.

During the 1990s, more functional temporary spacers were developed that incorporate small metallic femoral runners and polyethylene inserts into molded polymethylmethacrylate components. One such device, the so-called **PROSTALAC** (prosthesis of antibiotic loaded acrylic cement) allows joint motion and weight bearing during the period prior to reimplantation.[6] A range of motion up to 75 degrees has been reported with the use of this temporary functional spacer.[6] In a similar manner, some surgeons have sterilized the extracted femoral component and reinserted it temporarily using a small polyethylene insert on a cement block.[7] Again, this can reduce the patient's disability between debridement and staged reimplantation. If an articulating spacer is used, then attention must be paid to equalizing the flexion and extension space or dislocation may occur.

Aspiration prior to reimplantation is considered if there is clinical suspicion of persistent infection. However, in most cases our decision to proceed with reimplantation is determined intraoperatively based upon the appearance of the tissues and an evaluation of histologic frozen section specimens. At the time of reimplantation, adequate surgical exposure must be obtained and use of one of the previously discussed techniques, such as the quadriceps snip, may be required. Although uncemented prostheses with bone graft soaked in antibiotic solution have been used successfully in reimplantation,[8] we favor the use of cemented prostheses. The use of antibiotic-impregnated cement at the time of reimplantation has been shown to be associated with a significantly lower risk of recurrent infection.[9]

Significant bone loss, which requires the use of modular wedges or blocks, is often encountered at the time of reimplantation. Therefore, a prosthesis system, which has a full range of modular augments and stem extensions, should be available at reimplantation. The use of stemmed components does not necessarily require that a fully constrained articulation be implanted. Rather, the use of more constrained designs are reserved for cases with ligamentous insufficiency or instability. In the majority of reimplantations we recurrently use a cemented posterior stabilized prosthesis. We prefer to cement only the core prosthesis and avoid introduction of cement into the canal when stem extensions are used. This facilitates removal of the stems if subsequent prosthesis removal is required. In very rare cases with severe bone loss, custom prostheses or modular tumor prostheses may be required; the need for these devices must be anticipated preoperatively.

The postoperative management of individual patients is dependent on numerous variables, including the status of the soft tissue coverage, the type of exposure required, and whether structural bone grafts were utilized. In general, antibiotics are administered intravenously until final intraoperative culture results and tissue section evaluations have been obtained. If all results are negative for infection, then antibiotics are discontinued.

CLINICAL RESULTS

Insall originally reported on the successful eradication of infected total knee replacements with the two-stage protocol in 1977.[2] Windsor et al later confirmed the success of this technique when they reported on 38 reimplantations with an average follow-up of 4 years.[4] The two-stage protocol successfully eradicated the original deep infection in 37 knees (97.4%) and the reinfection rate was 10.5% (4 of 38 knees). Goldman reported on the largest cohort of two-stage reimplantations for infection.[1] The 64 knees in this study had an average follow-up of 7.5 years. Six knees (9%) became infected after reimplantation. With only two reinfections with the same organism, the infection eradication rate (97%) was identical to the findings of Windsor.[4]

Infection after total knee replacement is a serious and potentially devastating complication. Successful treatment can be obtained with the two-stage protocol. The long-term functional results, reinfection rate, and survivorship are comparable with those of revision total knee replacement.[1]

References
1. Goldman RT, Scuderi GR, Insall JN. Two-stage reimplantation for infected total knee replacement. *Clin Orthop.* 1996; 331:118–124.

2. Insall JN, Thompson FM, Brause BD. Two-stage reimplantation for the salvage of infected total knee arthroplasty. *J Bone Joint Surg*. 1983; 65A:1087–1098.

3. Windsor RE, Bono JV. Infected total knee replacements. *J Am Acad Orthop Surg*. 1994; 2:44–53.

4. Windsor RE, Insall JN, Urs WK, et al. Two-stage reimplantation for the salvage of total knee arthroplasty complicated by infection. Further follow-up and refinement of indications. *J Bone Joint Surg*. 1990; 72A: 272–278.

5. Booth RE, Jr, Lotke PA. The results of spacer block technique in revision of infected total knee arthroplasty. *Clin Orthop*. 1989; 248:57–60.

6. Masri BA, Kendall RW, Duncan CP, et al. Two-stage exchange arthroplasty using a functional antibiotic-loaded spacer in the treatment of the infected knee replacement: The Vancouver experience. *Sem. Arthroplasty*. 1994;5(3):122–136.

7. Hofmann AA, Kane KR, Tkach TK, Plaster RL, Camargo MP. Treatment of infected total knee arthroplasty using an articulating spacer. *Clin Orthop*. 1995; 321:45–54.

8. Whiteside LA. Treatment of infected total knee arthroplasty. *Clin Orthop*. 1994; 299:169–172.

9. Hanssen AD, Rand JA, Osmon DR. Treatment of the infected total knee arthroplasty with insertion of another prosthesis: The effect of antibiotic-impregnated bone cement. *Clin Orthop*. 1994; 309:44–55.

Chapter 12
Acute and Chronic Rupture of the Quadriceps Tendon Treated with Direct Repair

Robert E. Booth and Frank P. Femino

Rupture of the quadriceps tendon after total knee arthroplasty is rare and there is scant information in the literature regarding this problem.[1-3] In the nonimplant population, quadriceps tendon rupture is the more common malady in the older patient and patellar tendon rupture in the younger patient.[4-6] The reverse seems to be true after knee replacement despite the older average age of this population.

The causes of quadriceps rupture in the total knee arthroplasty patient are multiple. They include mechanical, systemic, and local factors. Mechanically, the tensile forces generated across the quadriceps tendon are very high, with values approaching 3000 newtons. They are greater than the forces in the patellar tendon at 90 and 120 degrees of flexion but less at 60 degrees of flexion.[7] In the setting of soft tissue compromise and with such large forces being sustained by the extensor mechanism, it is not surprising that rupture of the quadriceps tendon can occur after a total knee arthroplasty. Vascular and soft tissue compromise following surgical procedures such as a lateral retinacular release or a Roux-Goldthwaite procedure can lead to rupture and several cases have also been reported.[2,3]

In a patient with a total knee arthroplasty there is little contraindication to directly repairing the acutely ruptured quadriceps tendon. If there is minimal soft tissue compromise, the techniques used in nonarthroplasty patients are perfectly valid. These techniques are widely described in the literature and include end-to-end repair alone or with supplemental fixation.[4,5,8] The problem arises when, as is often the case in the total knee arthroplasty patient, there is structural compromise of the quadriceps tendon. This can make re-rupture common. Whether the rupture is acute or chronic often makes little difference. Therefore, reinforcement of the repair and augmentation of the soft tissue is advised. Techniques are described using various reinforcement techniques such as a quadriceps turndown flap (Fig. 12.1, Scuderi turndown technique).[6,9] In the chronic situation, the Codivilla technique of quadriceps lengthening may be necessary due to shortening of the extensor mass (Fig. 12.2, Codivilla technique of tendon lengthening and repair).[10]

The results for early repair of acute quadriceps tendon ruptures in nonarthroplasty patients have been excellent.[4,11] The functional outcome in the patient with a total knee arthroplasty has been consistently inferior. Extensor lag and quadriceps weakness are common and may require bracing.[1,2,12] The repair should be protected for several months.[1,3] A series of three repairs reported by Lynch and colleagues resulted in one re-rupture after 6 weeks, leaving a 35-degree permanent extension lag, as well as limited flexion and significant extension lag in the other two.[3] The only

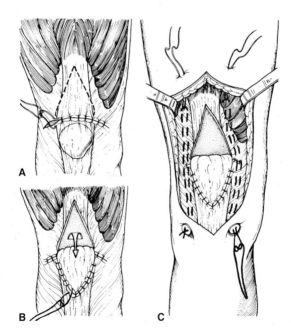

FIGURE 12.1. The Scuderi technique for repairing acute tears of the quadriceps tendon. (A) The torn edges of the quadriceps tendon are debrided and repaired. (B) A triangular flap of the proximal tendon is developed, folded distally over the rupture, and sutured in place. (C) Pullout sutures are then placed in the medial and lateral retinaculum.

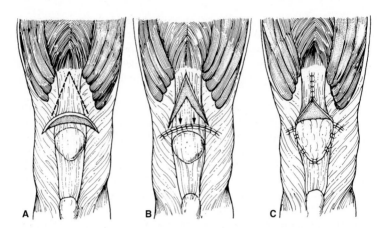

FIGURE 12.2. The Codvilla quadriceps tendon lengthening and repair for chronic ruptures. (A) The torn tendon edges are debrided and repaired. (B) An inverted V is cut through the proximal tendon. (C) The flap is brought distally and sutured in place. The upper portion on the V defect is then repaired.

exception is a case reported by Fernandez-Baillo and associates[13] in which he repaired a traumatic rupture of the quadriceps tendon occurring over 1 month after a total knee replacement. He used the technique described by Scuderi and reinforced the repair with Dacron tape. The functional result was good after 1 year, with no pain, a range of motion of 0 to 110 degrees, and almost normal quadriceps strength.[13]

It is our recommendation to perform the repair as soon as possible, because acute repair will minimize further quadriceps atrophy and shortening. We prefer the technique as described by Scuderi with the discretionary use of Dacron tape reinforcement, based on intraoperative assessment. Postoperative treatment consists of full weight-bearing in a cylinder cast for 6 weeks. The cast is then removed and gradual flexion is begun in a protective hinged brace. Physical therapy for strengthening is started. Our goal is to reach 90 degrees of flexion at 3 months with minimal extensor lag. Maximum results can be expected between 6 and 12 months.

References

1. Gustillo RB, Thompson R. Quadriceps and patellar tendon ruptures following total knee arthroplasty. In: Rand JA, Dorr LD, eds. *Total Arthroplasty of the Knee*. Rockville, Maryland: Aspen, 1987:45.

2. Doolittle KH, Turner RH. Patellofemoral problems following total knee arthroplasty. *Orthop Rev.* 1988; 17:696–702.

3. Lynch AF, Rorabeck CH, Bourne RB. Extensor mechanism complications following total knee arthroplasty. *J Arthroplasty.* 1987; 2:135–140.

4. Siwek CW, Rao JO. Ruptures of the extensor mechanism of the knee joint. *J Bone Joint Surg.* 1981; 63A:932–937.

5. Larsen E, Lund PM. Ruptures of the extensor mechanism of the knee joint. *Clin Orthop.* 1986; 213:150–153.

6. Murzic WJ, Hardaker WT, Goldner JL. Surgical repair of extensor mechanism ruptures of the knee. *Complic Orthop.* 1992; 7:276–279.

7. Huberti HH, Hayes WC, Stone JL, Shybut GT. Force ratios in the quadriceps tendon and ligamentum patellae. *J Orthop Res.* 1984; 2: 49–54.

8. Walker LG, Glick H. Bilateral spontaneous quadriceps tendon ruptures. *Orthop Rev.* 1989; 18:867–871.

9. Scuderi C. Ruptures of the quadriceps tendon. *Am J Surg.* 1958; 95: 626–634.

10. Scuderi C, Schrey EL. Ruptures of quadriceps tendon; study of 14 tendon ruptures. *Arch Surg.* 1950; 61:42–54.

11. Rasul AT, Fischer DA. Primary repair of quadriceps tendon ruptures. *Clin Orthop.* 1993:205–207.

12. MacCollum MS, Karpman RR. Complications of the PCA anatomic patella. *Orthopedics.* 1989; 12:1423–1428.

13. Fernandez-Baillo N, Garay EG, Ordonez JM. Rupture of the quadriceps tendon after total knee arthroplasty: a case report. *J Arthroplasty.* 1993:331–333.

Chapter 13

Management of Patella Tendon Disruptions in Total Knee Arthroplasty

Giles R. Scuderi and Brian C. De Muth

Extensor mechanism disruptions are an unwelcome complication of primary and especially revision total knee arthroplasty. Management of these disruptions can be extremely challenging, and often fraught with disappointing results. While the previous chapter addressed quadriceps disruptions, this chapter will focus on management of patella tendon disruptions in total knee arthroplasty.

Without question, the optimal method of management for extensor mechanism disruptions in total knee arthroplasty is to avoid them. Even though several types of extensor mechanism repairs will be discussed herein, none can offer results comparable to a repair that is not needed. Therefore, every possible effort should be made to prevent them. This is especially important to bear in mind when planning a TKR for a patient with increased risk for extensor mechanism complications. Those at high risk include patients who are obese, have poor preoperative motion, have had prior surgery about the tibial tubercle or patella tendon, have a connective tissue disorder, or have other metabolic conditions that may compromise their soft tissues.

TIBIAL TUBERCLE AVULSION

Tibial tubercle avulsions are perhaps the most common extensor mechanism disruptions encountered during total knee arthroplasty. Insall has previously described avulsions of the tibial tubercle as *"an intraoperative complication that should be avoided rather than treated."*[1] This point is reinforced by the paucity of documented successes in managing tibial tubercle avulsions once they do occur.[2-5] Therefore, great care should be taken intraoperatively to protect the attachment of the patella tendon to the tibial tubercle.

Three specific preventive measures to avoid this pitfall include:[1]

1. *Protect the tubercle at its insertion site.* Tension from the quadriceps mechanism above can cause the tendon to avulse by tearing across the periosteum, making adequate repair tenuous at best. This can be avoided by bringing the arthrotomy incision for initial exposure medial to the tibial tubercle and then raising a cuff of periosteum up to the tubercle. In tight knees in which exposure is difficult, the reflection of periosteum can be extended laterally with sharp vertical dissection to include up to 40% of the tubercle without significant loss of structural integrity of the extensor mechanism. This creates a "peel" of disection rather than a problematic transverse tear. If the tubercle does begin to avulse, a soft tissue sleeve is preserved that can be later repaired to the medial soft tissue envelope.

2. *Extend proximal exposure when needed.* Several means of enhancing exposure proximally have been described and are reviewed elsewhere in this text. These measures will help to protect the patella tendon attachment distally. The original quadriceps turndown as described by Coonse and Adams[5] has been subsequently modified to become an expansion of a standard medial parapatellar arthrotomy. The proximal apex of the arthrotomy is extended in "inverted-V" fashion by releasing the vastas lateralis distally and laterally until the patella can be adequately everted. The limitation of this exposure approach is the prolonged postoperative rehabilitation that must be observed. The "quadriceps snip" as described by Insall[1] is a more versatile modification that simply extends the quadriceps tendon incision proximally and laterally at an oblique angle. This simple technique is sufficient the majority of the time to allow for adequate exposure. In those instances when the patellar tendon insertion is still under considerable tension, the quadriceps snip can be combined with a lateral retinacular release to afford an even greater exposure. The quadriceps snip release is repaired with the arthrotomy at wound closure. The major advantage of the quadriceps snip is that it allows for immediate motion postoperatively and avoids the problems of extensor lag often seen with the Coonse-Adams release.[1]

3. *Osteotomize the tibial tubercle if necessary.* If all previous measures to enhance exposure still do not afford adequate exposure, traumatic avulsion can still be avoided. It is far better to raise the tibial tubercle with a large wedge of tibial bone to allow for reattachment with wires or screws. Although some authors have reported excellent results with this method,[6,7] others have reported complications at a disappointingly high frequency.[8] Familiarity with the proper technique avoids complication.

RUPTURE OF THE PATELLAR TENDON

Rupture of the patellar tendon after total knee replacement is a rare and typically devastating problem (Fig. 13.1). Unfortunately, the results of several methods of acute repair are almost uniformly poor.[2–4,9]

Numerous theories have been postulated to explain the etiology of late rupture of the patellar tendon following TKA. As mentioned previously, improper surgical technique that malaligns the knee or the position of any single component can play a contributory role. Some authors have found its occurrence more common in knees with limited motion.[10,11] Others have suggested impingement of the prosthesis on the patella tendon to blame.[12] Still others believe that compromise of the vascular supply to the patellar tendon is a critical component of its failure.[12,13]

The time of occurrence of post-arthroplasty patellar tendon rupture has been debated in the literature. In the series reported

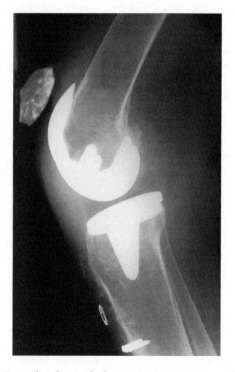

FIGURE 13.1. Lateral radiograph demonstrating a rupture of the patellar tendon, which is readily identified by the high riding patella.

by Cambi and Engh,[10] six of eight ruptures occurred intraoperatively or soon afterwards. In contrast, Gustillo and Thompson found most of the patellar tendon ruptures in their series to occur later.[4] Regardless of when the disruption occurs, no difference in management has been suggested to be time dependent.

Several repair techniques for patellar tendon disruption have been described. However, because the numbers in all post-arthroplasty case series have been low, no single technique can be considered a gold standard.

Predictably disappointing results have been noted with prolonged cast or brace immobilization alone as the sole means of management. This method of treatment may be adequate for partial tears, but the definitive diagnosis of an incomplete lesion is often difficult and not readily recognized. Therefore, open surgical repair is the preferred treatment. Reconstruction options include direct surgical repair, local autologous graft, distant autologous graft, synthetic graft, or various types of allograft.

Complete acute tendon tears may be managed with direct repair, but will most likely need some method of augmentation. In order to maximize the effectiveness of the repair and minimize ensuing stiffness, the repair should be carried out as soon as possible. If the tear occurs in the mid portion of the tendon, an end-to-end repair technique may be employed. Several means of enhancing the suture fixation during direct repair have been described including a Bunnell suture weave,[7] or a tendon grabbing stitch. The tendon should be repaired with nonabsorbable suture materials and, if present, the paratenon closed with absorbable sutures. Unfortunately, mid-tendon tears are less common than tears near the tendon origin or insertion. These later injuries are far more difficult to treat.

Bony avulsion or patellar tendon tears at the inferior pole of the patella are best managed by a traditional Bunnell-type repair with sutures passed through drill holes at the apex of the patella. It is important to reproduce the original length of the patella tendon when tensioning the sutures. Patella position can be ensured by comparing measurement of tendon length or position on a lateral radiograph with the opposite knee. Patellar baja must be avoided. Many authors also recommend a reinforcing cerclage suture encircling the tibial tubercle and the quadriceps tendon to protect the repair postoperatively. It would be our preference to use a #5 nonabsorbable suture rather than a metallic wire. Postoperative rehabilitation protocols vary. Typically, however, the knee is kept in full extension for 4 to 8 weeks with quadriceps setting exercise begun immediately. After allowing adequate time for soft tissue healing (approximately 6 weeks), the knee is started on a progressive range-of-motion and strengthening program. Unrestricted weight-bearing and flexion activities are permitted at about 12 weeks.

Tendon tears in close proximity to the tibial tubercle insertion pose a far greater repair challenge. A similar scenario occurs when the integrity of the distal remains of the patellar tendon is inadequate for a secure repair. In these clinical settings, the surgeon must choose between one of several reconstructive procedures. Unfortunately, large clinical series that establish the efficacy of any one technique do not exist.

One of the earliest described repair techniques for a patellar tendon-deficient knee was described by Kelikian[14] (Fig. 13.2). He utilized the semitendinosus tendon by harvesting the proximal extent of the tendon up to the musculotendinous junction while

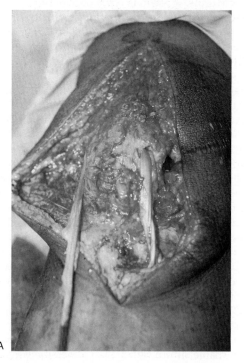

A

FIGURE 13.2. The semitendinosis tendon is passed through a transverse drill hole in the patella (A) and is sutured in place along the border of the patellar tendon (B).

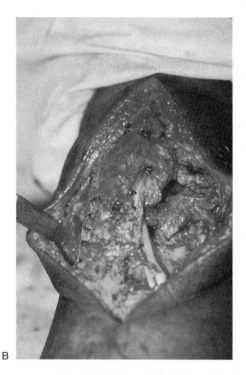

B

FIGURE 13.2. *Continued.*

leaving the distal insertion site intact. The freed proximal end of the tendon was then routed through holes drilled in the tibial tubercle and the patella before being secured back onto itself near its insertion site. If there is insufficient length, the gracilis tendon can also be harvested, detached, and sutured to the semitendinosis tendon. Ecker and associates[15] described a modification of this technique employing skeletal traction with a Steinmann pin through the superior pole of the patella to regain length of the shortened tendon. However, this technique is not recommended when a total knee replacement is present.

A modification of the Kelikian technique was reported by Cadambi and Engh[10] (Fig. 13.2). In a series of seven patients with a patellar tendon rupture following total knee replacement, the semitendinosus tendon was routed along the border of the remnant of the patellar tendon and then through a transverse hole in the inferior pole of the patella, anterior to the patellar implantbone interface. In two of their seven patients, the repair was augmented by harvesting the gracilis tendon and passing it through the patella drill hole as well. Postoperatively, weight-bearing was begun within 48 hours in a knee immobilizer or cast. Knee motion was then initiated at 6 weeks and progressed slowly over the next 10 weeks in a hinged knee brace. They reported that quadriceps strength and knee motion was restored in all patients.

Other authors have reported the successful use of allografts to manage disruptions of the extensor mechanism. Emerson and associates[3] have published on the successful use of an extensor mechanism allograft in a series of 15 patients with a rupture of the patella tendon in association with a total knee arthroplasty. The allograft consisted of the tibial tubercle, patellar tendon, patella, and quadriceps tendon that was freeze-dried or fresh-frozen. The graft was secured to the tibia with two screws distally and by non-absorbable suture attachment to native quadriceps tendon proximally. Motion was begun postoperatively as soon as the wound was sealed limiting flexion to 60 degrees in a hinged knee brace for the first 6 weeks, and progressed to 90 degrees by the end of the second 6 weeks. The authors reported that all but three patients received full active extension, with 66% of patients having no appreciable extensor lag.

More recently, Zanotti and colleagues[16] have reported successful treatment of a patellar tendon-deficient knee in a single patient with the use of a bone-patellar tendon-bone allograft. Their technique employed an irradiated, freeze-dried patellar-patellar tendon-proximal tibial allograft from a fresh cadaver. The host patella was prepared to accept the graft by creating a bone-to-bone interference fit further secured by circumferential sutures. The host tibia was prepared to accept the bone block of the graft, then tibial fixation was secured with a cortical screw. The repair was protected postoperatively in a cast for 3 months, and progressed to ambulation with a KAFO orthosis. They reported the graft to be healed with full active extension at 2-year follow-up.

Our current technique for reconstruction of chronic tears of the patellar tendon utilizes fresh-frozen extensor mechanism allograft that includes the tibial tubercle, patellar tendon, patella, and quadriceps tendon (Fig. 13.3). This is our preference because of the substantial amount of tissue that is available. Because disruptions of the extensor mechanism can lead to flexion instability, it is desirable to use a posterior-stabilized prosthesis. If there is any doubt about stability, then the arthroplasty should be revised to a constrained prosthesis. This may require revision of all the components. Finally, in planning the reconstruction, consideration must be given to the skin and surrounding soft tissues. It is not unusual

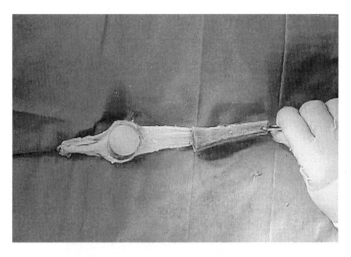

FIGURE 13.3. The extensor mechanism allograft.

to be referred a case for allograft reconstruction that has had several prior attempts at repair. Because the skin may be adherent or there may be multiple scars, soft tissue expanders have been shown to be helpful, and should be considered.[12] This is also important because the tibial tubercle allograft does add bulk to the proximal tibia making closure difficult.

TECHNIQUE
Following exposure of the knee, it is preferred to maintain the residual patellar tendon and surrounding fibrous tissue, because this provides a vascular tissue layer for later closure over the allograft. If the femoral and tibial components require revision, it is best to perform this step prior to placement of the allograft. Any hardware about the tibial tubercle should be removed. Whether to resurface the patella allograft remains debatable. It is our current preference not to resurface the patella.

The tibia is prepared by creating a trough about 60 to 80 mm long, which is fashioned along the tibial tubercle and tibial crest. The trough is created by removing the anterior cortex and compressing the underlying cancellous bone. Distally the osteotomy should be oblique in order to reduce the stress riser. Additionally, if possible, a rim of cortical bone should be maintained beneath the tibial component. The allograft then can be "keyed" into place (Fig. 13.4).

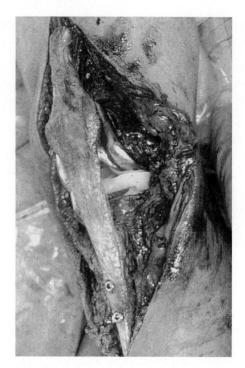

FIGURE 13.4. The extensor allograft in place.

At this point, the patella height needs to be determined in order to set the position of the tibial bone graft. With the knee in full extension, the patella should sit over the anterior flange of the femoral component and the inferior border of the patella approximately 1 cm above the joint line. Once the patella position is selected, the tibial bone graft is secured either with two bicortical screws or two cerclage wires. If the tibial component is being revised, the cerclage wires should be passed through drill holes in the tibial diaphysis and placed posterior to the tibial stem. With a stem extension in place, it may be difficult to set the screws or pass the wires.

The allograft quadriceps tendon is then passed through a transverse slit in the host quadriceps tendon. With the knee in full extension, the quadriceps tendon allograft is secured to the quadriceps expansion with multiple nonabsorbable sutures. The original patella is thinned to a wafer, or cortical shell. A patellectomy is not performed because the residual patella bone facilitates healing and serves as a useful landmark. It usually sits over the patella allograft and makes an interesting postoperative radiograph because two patellae can be seen (Fig. 13.5).

At this point, the range of motion and tension are checked. The range of motion is usually 45 to 60 degrees of flexion, and if properly oriented, the patella tracks centrally without a tilt. While the medial quadriceps retinaculum is sutured to the medial margin of the allograft, the lateral retinacular release is left open. The knee is then closed in a routine fashion and immobilized in extension with a cast or brace for 6 weeks. During this time the patient is allowed to ambulate full weight-bearing and encouraged to practice quadriceps setting exercises. After 6 weeks, the knee is braced and gradual range-of-motion exercises are initiated. The brace is discontinued when there is radiographic evidence that the tibial bone graft is healed, and the quadriceps muscle power is difficult to support the leg.

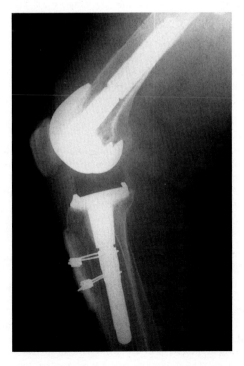

FIGURE 13.5. Postoperative radiograph showing the extensor allograft in place. Note the double patella.

Our clinical experience with this reconstruction technique includes six cases of extensor mechanism allografts for chronic rupture of the patellar tendon. Although four patients have full active extension, there are two patients who have an extensor lag less than 10 degrees. The average knee flexion is 90 degrees. All six patients are ambulating independently.

References

1. Insall JN, Haas SB. Complications of total knee arthroplasty, In: Insall JN. *Surgery of the Knee*. New York: Churchill Livingstone; 1993: 891–934.
2. Doolittle KH, Turner RH. Patellofemoral problems following total knee arthroplasty. *Orthop Rev*. 1988; 17:696–671.
3. Emerson RH, Head WC, Manlinin TI. Extensor mechanism reconstruction with an allograft after total knee arthroplasty. *Clin Orthop*. 1994; 303:79–85.
4. Gustillo RB, Thompson R. Quadriceps and patellar tendon ruptures following total knee arthroplasty. In: Rand JA, Dorr LD, eds. *Total Arthroplasty of the Knee*. Rockville, Maryland: 1987: 41–47.
5. Coonse K, Adams JD. A new operative approach to the knee joint. *Surg Gynecol Obstet*. 1943; 77:344–347.
6. MacCollum RF, Karpman RR. Complications of the PCA anatomica patella. *Orthopedics*. 1989; 12:1423–1429.
7. Sewik CW, Rao JO. Ruptures of the extensor mechanism of the knee joint. *J Bone Joint Surg*. 1981; 63A:932–937.
8. Whiteside LA, Ohl MD. Tibial tubercle osteotomy for exposure of the difficult total knee arthroplasty. *Clin Orthop*. 1990; 260:6–9.
9. Matava M. Patella tendon ruptures. *J Am Acad Orthop Surg*. 1996; 4:287–296.
10. Cadambi A, Engh GA. Use of a semitendinosus autogenous graft for rupture of the patellar ligament after total knee arthroplasty. *J Bone Joint Surg*. 1992; 74A:974–979.
11. Rand JA, Morrey BF, Bryan RS. Patella tendon ruptures after total knee arthroplasty. *Clin Orthop*. 1989; 224:233.
12. Gold DA, Scott WN. Soft tissue expansion prior to arthroplasty in the multiply-operated knee. A new method of preventing catastrophic skin problems. *J Arthroplasty*. 1996; 11(5):512–521.
13. Laskin RS. Total condylar knee replacement in rheumatoid arthritis. *J Bone Joint Surg*. 1981; 69A:29.
14. Kelikian H, Riashi E, Gleason J. Restoration of quadriceps function in neglected tear of the patella tendon. *Surg Gynecol Obstet*. 1957; 104: 200–204.
15. Ecker ML, Lotke PA, Glazer RM. Late reconstruction of the patella tendon. *J Bone Joint Surg*. 1979; 61A:884–886.
16. Zanotti RM, Freidberg AA, Mathews LS. Use of patellar allograft to reconstruct a patellar tendon-deficient knee after total joint arthroplasty. *J Arthroplasty*. 1995; 10(3):271–274.

Chapter 14
Revision of Periprosthetic Femur Fractures

Robert E. Booth and David G. Nazarian

Distal femoral fractures associated with a total knee arthroplasty are mercifully rare, as they are arguably among the most difficult osseous infractions to treat. Fractures occurring *outside* the "no-man's land" between the femoral epicondyles and the femoral diaphysis (some 12 cm proximal) are less problematic. Femoral diaphyseal fractures have good bone, less comminution, and sufficient distance from the joint to be minimally affected by the arthroplasty itself. Fractures distal to the femoral epicondyles do not involve the collateral ligaments of the knee, and they can be treated with simple revisional augmentations.

Periprosthetic total knee fractures within 3 to 15 mm of the joint line, however, hold several distinct hazards. First, they can occur with surprisingly little trauma to the limb yet with severe bony comminution. In fact, as a general rule, the less the trauma, the worse the fracture. This is explained by the second point, which is that the supracondylar area of the femur is extremely osteoporotic in these patients, with thin cortices and practically no intramedullary cancellous bone. Once the "eggshell" of the distal femur has cracked, reconstructive efforts will be frustrated by the simple lack of substance proximal to the arthroplasty.

Third, it is rarely appreciated that one of the contributing factors to the fracture is the unsatisfactory nature of the original arthroplasty. This is particularly true of stiff total knees, most commonly the result of a tight posterior cruciate ligament or oversized components. The stress that this stiff arthroplasty places on the femoral bone not only predisposes to fracture, but also confounds attempts at stable fixation. While one would prefer to treat either the fracture or the failed total joint individually, it is often necessary to address these problems simultaneously, since they are so interrelated.

For biologic as well as sociologic reasons, conservative treatment of supracondylar femoral fractures is almost impossible today, and open intervention of some variety is usually necessary.

Many techniques of internal fixation are available, but all share significant technical difficulties as well as a surprisingly high incidence of nonunion and malunion. The medial mechanical axis of the lower limb, the concerted action of the posterior knee musculature, and the sagittal plane of motion of the joint itself all conspire to destabilize even the most rigid internal fixation. This is compounded by the effects of bony comminution, severe femoral osteopenia, and a stiff knee arthroplasty. It is not surprising, therefore, that many fractures develop nonunions or go on to a tardy malunion with the typical deformity of adduction, flexion, and internal rotation of the distal femoral fragment.

Rush rod fixation, as espoused by Ritter[1] is economical and expeditious, but in most cases has provided insufficient stabilization. Better results have been found with distal condylar plate and screw devices,[2] although even good surgical results will often deteriorate into nonunion or malunion and the bone available for distal screw fixation is often compromised by the intercondylar design of the femoral prosthetic component. New plating systems with abundant supracondylar screw options may improve this situation, but the biologic issues of bone quality and joint dynamics will remain.

The competing principles of fracture immobilization in the face of joint mobility require ever more rigid fixation. The use of intramedullary rods, introduced through the intercondylar notch of most prostheses, is an attractive option that requires minimal disturbance of the arthroplasty. Excellent results have been reported with this technique,[3] although several important technical issues should be considered. First, the precise design of the prosthetic femoral component must be known, so that a rod of sufficient diameter to achieve intramedullary stabilization of the fracture can be introduced through the open box of the femoral component. The diameters of these components are well known (Table 14.1). There have been apocryphal reports of the need for a "prosthetic notch plasty" using a Midas Rex burr to enlarge the metallic intercondylar space, although this is clearly not to be recommended.

Second, one should be prepared for the necessity to open the fracture site above the femoral prosthesis and place an intercalary allograft—sculpted from a distal femur—to surround the intramedullary rod, fill the metaphyseal void, maintain femoral limb length, and provide support for the comminuted host cortical bone, which can be wired about the graft. Without this graft material, the rod alone may be insufficient to maintain length and promote healing of the fracture. Finally, one may enhance the function of the stiff arthroplasty after stabilization of the fracture by

TABLE 14.1. Intercondylar distances of commonly used total knee implants*

Implant	Intercondylar distance (mm)
Miller-Galante (Zimmer, Warsaw, IN)	12
Insall-Burstein (Zimmer)	14–19
Biomet (Warsaw, IN)	22
Intermedics (Austin, TX)	18
AMK (DePuy, Warsaw, IN)	14–17
Osteonics (Allendale, NJ)	19
PFC (Johnson & Johnson, New Brunswick, NJ)	20
Kirschner wires (Timonium, MD)	20
Genesis (Smith & Nephew Richards, Memphis, TN)	20
Duracon (Howmedica, Rutherford, NJ)	12–16

*Reproduced, with modification, from: Engh and Ammen[4]

sectioning an excessively tight posterior cruciate ligament or downsizing an excessively thick patellar button.

All too frequently, none of these options will suffice. The total knee arthroplasty may be too bad to salvage, compromising the fracture healing and yielding a dysfunctional limb even if union should occur. The "personality" of the fracture may be unattractive, with such problems as profound comminution, insufficient distal bone for screw or rod fixation, periprosthetic bone loss secondary to prefracture osteolysis, or intercondylar fragmentation and compromise of collateral support. In these and other severe situations, simultaneous revision of the arthroplasty and stabilization of the fracture must be considered. This can be a heroic endeavor, to be undertaken only by those with a full array of revisional prostheses and tools, an adequate supply of allograft material, and extensive total knee revisional experience.

In the operating room, one must be prepared for an extended surgical procedure, with sufficient anesthetic to last several hours. Some thighs will be too short to permit a proper tourniquet, although a sterile tourniquet can be used to maintain hemostasis through much of the procedure. The preferred incision is an extension of the knee arthrotomy midline incision well up into the proximal thigh. This approach will even allow the removal of prior failed fixation devices from the medial or lateral side of the femur without the use of parallel skin incisions. All prior prosthetic materials must be removed, and it is generally preferable to address the previous fracture materials before removing the femoral component of the total knee. This will protect the fragile distal femoral bone as long as possible during the surgery.

The optimal stabilization of the fracture usually involves a long intramedullary rod, extending several inches at least above the fracture site. This must be compatible with the new total knee arthroplasty and systems such as the constrained condylar knee remain the industry standard. Curved rods may be necessary to match the femoral bow, and they have the additional advantage of conferring some rotational stability upon the ultimate construct. Rods of 150 to 200 mm of length are most helpful. Offset rods may additionally allow for accommodation of previous fracture malunions.

The mechanism of failure of the index arthroplasty must be clearly understood and reversed. Most frequently this involves conversion from a cruciate retaining to a cruciate substituting design, downsizing of prosthetic components, and correction of internal rotational malalignment of the femoral and tibial components. Extra hands are often needed during surgery even to place trial components, since the distal femoral fragment in particular will be difficult to control, tending to flex and internally rotate in response to muscle influences about the knee.

Once a prosthetic device has been selected and trials implanted, the fracture can be addressed. Particular attention should be paid to the proper rotation of the limb, often using palpation of the posterior linea aspera to confirm position. Whether fresh fracture, malunion, or nonunion, the interface between the proximal and femoral and distal femoral fragments may need to be simplified and freshened. This is preferably performed in an oblique fashion, avoiding butt or step cuts. An oblique osteotomy provides greater bone surface for healing, partial correction of flexion deformities, and significant stability against rotation. Occasionally, supplemental cortical plating of the fracture may be necessary, although only unicortical screw fixation will be available if the intramedullary rod is of appropriate substance.

Extensive grafting of the fracture may be required. At the very least, small bone fragments or *paste* will be helpful at the termination of the procedure to enhance healing in an area of extreme osteopenia. An *intercalary graft*, fashioned to surround the intramedullary rod but provide bulk and fill for the supracondylar area may be extremely helpful, as previously described in the retrograde rodding technique. Occasionally, the distal bone is of such poor quality that an entire distal *femoral allograft* may be needed. An arthroplasty of the graft can be performed on a back table, then mated with the host femur within the operative field. The junction of the massive allograft can be accomplished either by invagination of the graft within the residual femoral canal or—as described previously—by an oblique osteotomy. In either situation, the graft surmounting the intramedullary rod should be made intentionally too long, then whittled to proper limb length once the arthroplasty has been balanced in flexion. This allows the secondary adjustment of proper extension balance in the same way that one would balance a simple revisional arthroplasty using prosthetic augments.

If an intercondylar fracture should occur during the procedure, the bony fragments should be preserved with their attached collateral ligaments. These can be cemented at the time of fracture reduction within the "pockets" of the femoral component, secured with methylmethacrylate and held temporarily by a bone clamp, potentially reinforced with mersilene tape. The medial collateral ligament is, of course, of the highest priority, since even a constrained condylar knee system will display rotational instability in its absence. Onlay cortical plates or struts may be wired about the host/graft junction to augment bone stock, contain residual cortical fragments, and confer further rotational stability. The late incorporation of these grafts is quite good, much as has been observed in proximal femoral hip reconstructions.

Finally, it is the obligation of the surgeon to confer stability upon both the fracture and the arthroplasty at the time of surgery. Occasionally, this may require cementation of the intramedullary stem. This should be done with caution because of potential future revisional difficulties as well as possible sequestration of some of the fracture fragments. Intramedullary rods appropriate for cementation should be used, as well as cement restrictors. Internal stabilization of these fractures is far preferable to subsequent external bracing, although this adjunctive therapy may be helpful in the early mobilization of some reconstructions. Protected weightbearing is at the discretion of the surgeon, influenced by the extent of the allograft, the stability of the reconstruction, the need for postoperative motion, and patient compliance.

When successful, simultaneous revision of an unsatisfactory knee arthroplasty and fixation of the fracture it precipitated can be an extremely satisfying and costeffective procedure.

References

1. Ritter MA, Keating EM, Faris PM, Meding JB. Rush rod fixation of supracondylar fractures above total knee arthroplasties. *J Arthroplasty.* 1995; 10:213–216.

2. Healy WL, Siliski JM, Incavo SJ. Operative treatment of distal femoral fractures proximal to total knee replacements. *J Bone Joint Surg.* 1993; 75-A:27–34.
3. Henry SL, Booth RE. Management of supracondylar fractures proximal to total knee arthroplasty with GSH supracondylar nail. *Contemp Orthop.* 1995; 31:231–238.
4. Engh GA, Ammeen DJ. Periprosthetic fractures adjacent to total knee implants. *J Bone Joint Surg.* 1997; 79-A:1100–1113.

Chapter 15
Revision Arthroplasty for Tibial Periprosthetic Fractures

Wayne G. Paprosky, Todd D. Sekundiak, and John Kronick

Despite the increasing number of total knee arthroplasties being performed,[1] the rate of periprosthetic tibial fractures has remained low. Healy performed a retrospective review of the English-language literature from 1970 to 1992 and found 32 reported cases in nine published articles.[2-11] These fractures are much less common than supracondylar femoral fractures with Cordeiro and associates reporting a relative ratio of nine to one.[4] Treatment options for these fractures have included a host of different operative and nonoperative techniques with revision arthroplasty being indicated in a select group.

No complete series of periprosthetic tibial fractures has been reported in the literature. The 15 tibial plateau fractures reported by Rand and Coventry[8] only included fractures that they felt were stress related from component malalignment or improper component rotation. It excluded fractures that occurred intraoperatively, secondary to trauma, or component failure. All fractures involved the medial plateau and were attributable to excessive medial displacement and varus positioning of the tibial component. This increased eccentric loading of the medial tibial plateau, in bone of poor quality and with a component that does not distribute force, led to resultant fracture.[12,13] These stress fractures had concomitant component loosening and required revision arthroplasty ultimately. Other authors have also correlated these stress fractures to component loosening and malalignment.[3,6,9,11]

These stress fractures have to be differentiated from fractures that occur from definitive trauma. As the prevalence of total knee arthroplasties increases in a younger more active population, periprosthetic tibial fracture from associated trauma will also increase. Treatment modalities will need to consider a host of variables, as with fracture management in general, to determine the most judicious approach. Traumatic injuries must be differentiated further by the amount of energy when determining treatment. High-energy fractures may preclude certain treatments secondary to the degree of bone and soft tissue loss, the higher risk of infection, the possibility of multiple or bilateral fractures, and the concern of multisystem injuries.

INCIDENCE

The incidence of periprosthetic tibial fractures has been reported at 1.7%.[8] This may actually be higher than that which exists because this rate has iatrogenic influence secondary to component malpositioning and selection. In Weidel's review of 800 total knee arthroplasties, no traumatic periprosthetic tibial fractures were found.[12] Bryan reported on 450 patients and reported a rate of 1%.[3] No difference has been found between control and fracture groups when body weight, duration of disease, disease of the contralateral lower extremity, or steroid use was compared.[8] Surprisingly, most series and case reports of periprosthetic tibial fractures occur from minimal trauma.[3–11] The most common presenting symptom is pain that can be present from 1 day to a year.[8] The delay in diagnosis is most commonly from the patient delaying medical advice.

TREATMENT OPTIONS

The goals with periprosthetic tibial fractures are similar to any particular fracture—to obtain fracture union with satisfactory limb alignment while maintaining ligamentous and tendinous tissue attachments and function. Chen and associates have proposed an algorithm for supracondylar femoral periprosthetic fractures that can be applied to tibial periprosthetic fractures.[15] Rand has also considered five factors in assessing the fracture character that determines an algorithm for treatment options. These are timing, location, and extent of the fracture, presence or absence of union, and the effect of the fracture on limb alignment as well as fracture alignment.[16] These then must be combined with host factors such as age, activity level, and concomitant systemic disease to determine treatment. Finally, consideration is given to the premorbid joint replacement that provides us with the following algorithm.

Most authors agree that with well-fixed, painless total knee arthroplasties, that union of a nondisplaced, stable fracture can be obtained with nonoperative measures secondary to the low-energy nature of these fractures.[17] Motion is preserved in a knee that has previously functioned well and has been casted for a short period to obtain union.[17]

For fractures that are displaced or unstable but occurring with a component that is well fixed and previously functioning well, there is controversy whether these should be treated open or closed—and if opened, if revision or internal fixation should proceed. Closed treatment should only be considered when reduction can be obtained and maintained. When closed treatment is not an option for a fracture because of the patient's inability to tolerate prolonged immobility or the surgeon's inability to reduce the fracture or maintain the alignment, open reduction and internal fixation is the next option.

Significant bone loss can occur with removal of previously well-fixed components, making revision arthroplasty indicated only when the soft tissue coverage, the previous implant and stem, or the fracture pattern precludes internal fixation. It is critical to summate the amount of bone loss that will occur from removal of the components, combined with the fracture pattern itself. Removal of components can extend the degree of comminution and must be considered with the patient's overall bone quality, to determine the type of prosthesis, stem, augmentation, and bone graft required. Further, it must be determined if it is technically feasible to reconstruct the joint immediately. It may be prudent to initially accept a malunion that allows bone stock and soft tissue coverage to improve with healing. Revision arthroplasty or osteotomy may then be easier and more effective than undertaking an immediate massive initial reconstruction that requires extensive resources to reconstruct an extremity with deficient bone and soft tissues.

The assessment of bone loss is even more critical when assessing a fracture with a component that is well-fixed but malpositioned. Because of the malpositioning of the component, one may feel obliged to revise the joint immediately. Ultimately all tibial periprosthetic stress fractures will require revision when they have occurred in the presence of a malpositioned component.[8] However, the revision procedure can be technically demanding and may be easier achieved once union has initially been obtained. If, however, stable fixation can be obtained with a revision arthroplasty without compromising significant host bone or soft tissues, then revision should be considered as the immediate definitive treatment.

In cases in which the component is loose, irrespective of the fracture being displaced or nondisplaced, revision arthroplasty is indicated. Some authors still initially seek union by closed treatment or internal fixation because reconstruction is fraught with hazards in the presence of a fresh fracture.[17] As stated previously, the technical demands of the reconstruction and the resources required will determine the timing of the reconstruction. Further caveats to this approach would be for patients unable to tolerate an operative procedure or where infection would be at high risk.

Nonunions, malunions, or delayed unions of tibial fractures can also be treated with a stemmed tibial revision component (Fig. 15.1). An established delayed or nonunion of the femur can be treated with internal fixation and bone grafting.[18] The periprosthetic tibia fracture, however, may have a tenuous soft tissue envelope that may lead to skin slough if one were to open the fracture site, graft, and obtain osteosynthesis. Open reduction and internal fixation of these fractures with plate osteosynthesis may also preclude future revision by encroachment of screws in the intramedullary canal. Placement of a stemmed component and use of intramedullary bone graft, for metaphyseal or diaphyseal fractures, can be used with great success as the fracture site is stabilized. Deformity is corrected. Motion of the joint can be maintained and the fracture site can be loaded (Fig. 15.1B).[19–21]

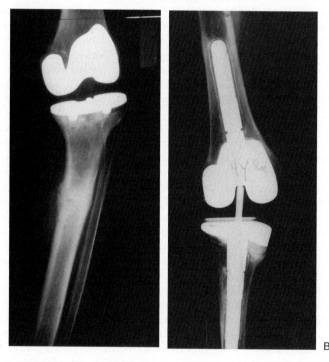

A   B

FIGURE 15.1. (A) Tibial nonunion with malpositioned uncemented components. (B) Revision arthroplasty at 4½ years. Nonunion has healed with stem bridging nonunion site. Joint deformity required metal augmentation to reconstruct joint line. Sclerotic halo around femoral stem is not indicative of failed component.

PREOPERATIVE PLANNING

The objectives in revision of total knee arthroplasty for ipsilateral periprosthetic tibial fractures are the same as for the principles of total knee arthroplasty. If revision arthroplasty is to be considered, preoperative planning must consider bone and soft tissue losses from traumatic and atraumatic causes—and the degree of deformity. Preoperative assessment includes full-length standing anteroposterior and lateral radiographs with magnification markers of the lower extremity. This provides accurate assessment of defect size, deformity angle, as well as component size, augment or stem length and width, and the need for an osteotomy. Treatment choices will be tempered not only by the noted anatomical deficits of the injury but also by the functional limitations or expectations of the patient. A custom long-stemmed tumor prosthesis can easily substitute for a comminuted metaphyseal fracture in an elderly debilitated patient, whereas a short-stemmed minimally constrained arthroplasty with limited internal fixation may function better for a younger active patient.

Removal of components, osteolysis, and osteopenia, in addition to the comminuted fracture fragments can significantly increase the amount of bone loss. This can necessitate the use of cement, bone graft, or augments in the revision procedure to fill defects. In instances in which severe bone loss or comminution exists, bulk structural allografting must be considered. Length and width of graft are measured, as well as the possible need for ligament and tendinous reconstruction (Fig. 15.2).

In the late setting of nonunions or malunions, angular deformities can be corrected in the metaphyseal region by bone resection or augmentation at the time of arthroplasty as long as the collateral ligaments or extensor mechanism is not compromised. Knowledge of ligamentous and tendinous insertions is essential and must be correlated to bony resection to determine if insertions will be compromised. For translational tibial deformities, offset tibial stems or baseplates with eccentric housing connections are useful for obtaining better tibial coverage without needing an osteotomy. Deformities that exist in the diaphyseal area of the tibia with greater than 10 to 15 degrees of angulation in the coronal plane or 20 degrees in the sagittal plane may require osteotomy and correction to perform a satisfactory arthroplasty.[16] To restore a normal mechanical axis, tracing paper outlining the deformity and resultant operative correction is used in deciding the method of correction.

Surgical exposure must be planned to include these adjunctive procedures of fracture fragment reduction, removal of old components or fixation devices, as well as new component insertion. If

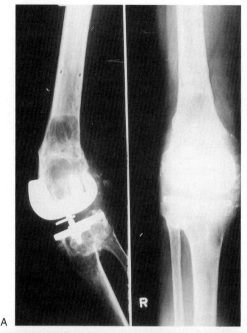

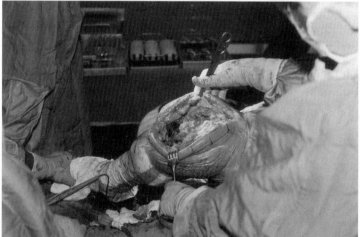

FIGURE 15.2. A 69-year-old male with severe osteolysis and fractures involving the medial femoral condyle and lateral tibial plateau. (A) Preoperative radiographs. (B) Tibial defect demonstrating severe loss of bone but integrity of tibial tubercle and extensor mechanism.

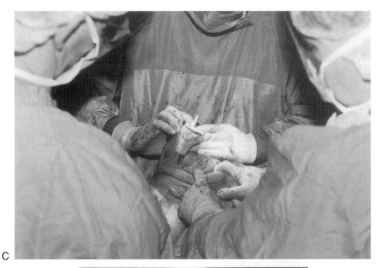

C

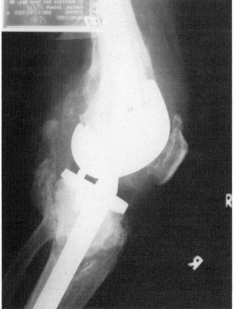

D

FIGURE 15.2. (C) Cemented tibial component and allograft press-fit in host bone. (D) Postoperative radiograph demonstrating graft invaginated in host bone with maintenance of host extensor mechanism.

possible, exposure should include previous operative incisions to prevent the possibility of skin ischemia and resultant slough.

Stemmed components have been indispensable adjuncts to these revision procedures. The use of stems in the revision setting has been discussed elsewhere. Most systems now have an array of fluted press-fit stems. Cemented stems have previously been used with great success but run the risk of nonunion by the presence of cement into the fracture site. For fractures that occur in the metaphyseal or diaphyseal region, the stem can be used like an intramedullary rod to bridge the fracture site and obtain rotational and bending stability (Fig. 15.1). For epiphyseal fractures, the stem can be used as an unloader to transmit force away from the joint and prevent collapse or migration of bony fragments after limited fixation, grafting, or removal of fragments has been performed (Fig. 15.3). The need for a constrained or nonconstrained

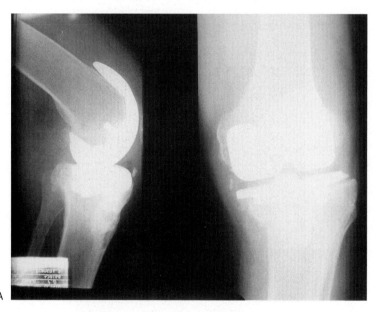

A

FIGURE 15.3. A 70-year-old male with two previous knee arthroplasties in two consecutive years. Patient began complaining of significant medial knee pain and sudden increasing deformity. (A) Preoperative radiograph demonstrating varus positioning of the tibial component with subsidence and fracturing of the medial tibial plateau.

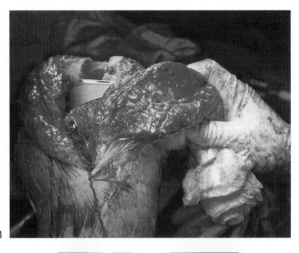

B

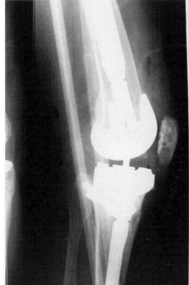

C

FIGURE 15.3. (B) Intraoperative photograph demonstrating lag screw fixation of medial tibial plateau fracture with stemmed component and augment then being positioned. (C) Postoperative radiograph of stemmed components. An offset stem was used to increase load on the intact lateral tibial plateau.

component is also determined. The compatibility of the stem to the type of component must also be considered because bridging a fracture with an intramedullary rod does not obligate the use of a constrained component.[19] Compatibility of the revision tibial stem and baseplate with the in situ femoral component must also be considered to determine the need and technical difficulty of its removal.

OPERATIVE TECHNIQUE

Revision knee arthroplasty for tibial periprosthetic fractures begins with an incision that must be extensile to allow adequate access to the knee for removal of components and for the possibility of exposure of fracture fragments. Tissues are compromised from previous operative procedures, but now also have the acute traumatic insult. Previous operative incisions must be incorporated as discussed elsewhere. Osteotomes or sliver osteotomes are routinely used for removal of well-fixed components. One needs to be cognizant of the force imparted on the arthroplasty interfaces because the force can be transmitted to the bone and lead to propagation of the fracture or fracture fragmentation. The use of a power saw or burr may remove some extra bone at the interface being debonded but avoids the peak forces that a mallet and osteotome may impart. This leads to a resultant increase in final bone stock integrity. Removal of components can proceed in a host of different ways but patience must be employed. Once component interfaces have been debonded, the components should be digitally pulled off the bone surfaces without the use of a mallet to expedite the removal.

With the components removed, the bone is curretted and cleansed to assess the bone defects present. In nearly all cases in which tibial component revision is the treatment for a periprosthetic fracture, a tibial intramedullary stem will be used to augment the component. This requires intramedullary alignment for the proximal tibial cut. The method of alignment is described elsewhere. Initially a minimal amount of proximal tibia is resected. "Clean-up" cuts are also performed on the femur, which then allows flexion and extension gaps to be assessed.

The presence of the fracture may prevent adequate assessment of the gaps at this time. If the fracture is metaphyseal or epiphyseal, then initial internal fixation should proceed. This will provide bony stability and then allow for assessment of ligamentous stability and flexion-extension gap balance. If fractures are metadiaphyseal or diaphyseal, fractures can be splinted with an intramedullary trial stem or guide rod that then allows the surgeon to place the appropriate strains to assess balance. Final cuts are then determined and made. Intramedullary reaming continues to accept the appropriate width and length of stem. Trial components are then placed and the joint reduced and moved through a range of motion. Final adjustments are made to accept the actual components.

Epiphyseal fractures or metaphyseal extensions of plateau fractures should be reduced and fixed to maintain as much host bone as possible and to help support the prosthesis. Screw or screw-and-plate fixation can be used as described by Schatzker with screw placement occurring to avoid possible impingement with an intramedullary revision stem or extension[22] (Fig. 15.3). Fixation should be stable but limited to avoid complications of the "dead bone sandwich." With revision arthroplasty being considered, stability will be augmented with stemmed components. If fracturing is limited to a small compression or split component, then metal base tray augmentation or small bulk allografting fixed with screws can be used to substitute for the defect.

The revision procedures for periprosthetic metaphyseal or diaphyseal tibial fractures, in which significant bone loss or comminution does not exist, proceed in a manner as previously described for revision knee arthroplasty but with a few modifications. If the fracture is metaphyseal, cementing the housing of the baseplate will provide stability to the proximal fracture fragment. A stem extension can then be press-fit into the diaphyseal bone to bridge the fracture and maintain alignment (Fig. 15.1). If the rod is being used to bridge the diaphyseal fracture site and not simply to protect epiphyseal fractured bone, intramedullary fixation occurs to a point approximately two to two-and-one-half diameters of the tibial shaft past the fracture site to allow for stability. Press-fitting of the rod occurs with reaming line-to-line. Reaming is slightly more aggressive than in routine revision with the aim of removing some endosteal cortical bone. This ensures cortical contact of the rod along a farther length of the endosteal cortical bone that gives stability to the fracture site in the bending and rotational planes.

Grafting of the fracture site to obtain union is indicated as for other fractures. Bone resected from the cut surfaces can occasionally be used as a structural graft but is indispensible in its morselized form for its osteoinductive potential. Its employment at the fracture site will also obviate the potential morbidity from another donor site. To improve stability and bone stock, morselized allogenic or autogenous bone can be impacted around the stem at the metaphyseal flare as previously described.[23] This grafting helps to control motion of the fracture site if it occurs at or proximal to the metaphyseal flare. Grafting will also support the tibial tray and provide a smoother transmission of joint forces to the host bone. When cementing the component in place, only the surface and housing of the component are cemented, ensuring that no cement intrudes at the fracture site.

Where proximal bone loss is significant or if the fracture is epiphyseal with significant comminution, use of a bulk structural allograft can be considered (Fig. 15.2). No series exists for periprosthetic fractures but has been described for salvage revisions or periarticular tumors.[24–26] A custom metaphyseal-replacing prosthesis can also be considered but cost and longevity of the system need to be realized. The allograft can replace the proximal bone that is missing or damaged. If loss extends past the tibial tubercle, then extensor mechanism reconstruction is required. Ligamentous replacement or possible reconstruction must also be considered with the use of constrained components. Alternatively a hinged prosthesis must be evaluated. The allograft can be sculpted to invaginate into the remaining host bone that may obviate the need for reconstruction of the soft tissues (Fig. 15.2B). Augmentation of the soft tissues can occur with screw or wire fixation from the host bone into the allograft.

The tibial component is sized to the allograft and cemented into the prepared allograft with an attached press-fit stem. Size of the stem is determined by reaming into the distal tibial intramedullary canal until adequate cortical chatter is felt and heard. With the use of fluted stems, fixation is usually stable in the bending and rotational planes so that no augmentation of fixation is required (Fig. 15.2B). Alternatively, a step cut at the host-graft junction can improve rotational stability. A transverse host-graft junction allows for final fine-tuning length adjustments while the stem is being impacted into the host. A transverse saw cut can also be trimmed for optimal contact at the host-graft interface. Plate fixation for rotational control is unnecessary and causes undo soft tissue stripping and furthers the risk of nonunion or soft tissue slough.

Tibial nonunions, delayed unions, or malunions are managed differently depending on the location of deformity. As discussed earlier, if the deformity is metaphyseal, then deformity can be corrected by performing the arthroplasty bone resections and augmenting further defects with metal or a small bulk allograft fixed with screws. The use of an offset stem or eccentric housing on a tibial baseplate allows for tibial coverage while maintaining mechanical alignment for those deformities that may be translational. Diaphyseal deformities require exposure of the site and debridement of the pseudoarthrosis or osteotomy of the malunion. Use of a guide rod and cannulated reamers passed across the deformity under fluoroscopy ensures that reaming is symmetric and that the deformity will be corrected with stem insertion.

Postoperative protocols include continuous passive motion for all patients with weight-bearing being dependent on the fracture configuration and stability of the implant. Stemmed tibial revisions that substitute for bone loss with metal augments or small bulk allografts can begin immediate weight-bearing as tolerated. Touch weight-bearing and bracing is used for a period of 3 to 6 months when bulk allografts are used. Weight-bearing is increased once graft union is seen.

RESULTS

Results and complications can be variable and dependent on the energy to cause the fractures and the type of reconstruction required. With the number of periprosthetic tibial fractures being small and with revision arthroplasty being reserved for a select group of patients, the success and complication rates for revision arthroplasty can only be estimated by extrapolation. For fractures with minimal bone loss and low energy, complication rates likely parallel other revision series. When fracturing is comminuted with severe bone loss, rates will likely parallel rates for complex allograft revisions for salvage procedures or tumor resection.[24] Overall, success of revision can be expected to be approximately 90% with 4- to 5-year follow-up if the fracture is uncomplicated.[15,20] Kress and associates reported on four tibial nonunions treated with knee arthroplasty and intramedullary rod fixation. All patients achieved union with 90 degrees of painfree motion.[20] However, if the fracture pattern necessitates structural allografting with the use of the revision component, complications vary from 36 to 85%[24–27] with results only being short term. Complications include infection, component dislocation, component loosening, refracturing, nonunion, muscle weakness, and tissue loss.[26] Union of the graft to the host will occur in 92 to 100% of the cases and satisfactory results averaging 90%.[27,28]

CONCLUSION

With the incidence of total knee arthroplasty increasing annually, the prevalence of active mobile patients will also increase. The low-energy stress fractures of the past will then be supplanted by high-energy complex fractures. This in addition to the fact that components are being implanted for ever-increasing durations will demand sound surgical algorithms to obtain optimal fracture treatment results. As with any long bone fracture, the first aim is to obtain fracture union with normal extremity alignment. The character of the fracture, with the functional and medical level of the patient, is combined with the status of the total knee arthroplasty to determine successful management. If this is not possible by closed or open means or not possible without significant morbidity to the patient, then revision arthroplasty for tibial periprosthetic fractures should be considered as a viable option.

References

1. Mendenhall S. Hip and knee implant review. *Orthopedic Network News.* 1995; 6:1–6.
2. Healy WL. Tibial fractures below total knee arthroplasty. In: *Current Concepts in Primary and Revision Total Knee Arthroplasty.* Lippincott-Raven; 1996:163–167.
3. Bryan RS, Peterson LFA, Combs JJ. Polycentric knee arthroplasty: a preliminary report of postoperative complications in 450 knees. *Clin Orthop.* 1973; 94:148–152.
4. Cordeiro EN, Costa RC, Carazzato JG, Silva J. Periprosthetic fractures in patients with total knee arthroplasties. *Clin Orthop.* 1990; 252:182–189.
5. Kjaersgaard-Andersen P, Juhl M. Ipsilateral traumatic supracondylar femoral and proximal tibial fractures following total knee replacement: a case report. *J Trauma.* 1989; 29:398–400.
6. Lotke PA, Ecker ML. Influence of positioning of prosthesis in total knee replacement. *J Bone Joint Surg Am.* 1977; 59:77–79.
7. Makela EA. Capacitively coupled electrical field in the treatment of a leg fracture after total knee replacement. *J Orthop Trauma.* 1992; 6:237–240.
8. Rand JA, Coventry MB. Stress fractures after total knee arthroplasty. *J Bone Joint Surg Am.* 1980; 62:226–233.
9. Skolnick MD, Brian RS, Peterson LFA, Combs JJ, Ilstrup DM. Polycentric total knee arthroplasty: a two year follow-up study. *J Bone Joint Surg Am.* 1976; 58:743–748.
10. Tietjens BR, Cullen JC. Early experience with total knee replacement. *NZ Med J.* 1975; 82:42–45.
11. Wilson FC, Venters GC. Results of knee replacement with the Walldius prosthesis: an interim report. *Clin Orthop.* 1976; 120:39–46.
12. Wiedel JD. Management of fractures around total knee replacement. In: *Total Knee Arthroplasty: A Comprehensive Approach.* Williams & Wilkins; 1984:258–267.
13. Haemmerle J, Bartel D, Chao E. Mechanical analysis of polycentric tibial tract loosening. Read at the Joint Applied Mechanics, Fluids Engineering and Bioengineering Conference. New Haven, Connecticut, June 15–17, 1977.

14. Nogi J, Caldwell JW, Kauzlarich JJ, Thompson RC. Load testing of geometric and polycentric total knee replacements. *Clin Orthop.* 1976; 114:235–242.

15. Chen F, Mont MA, Bachner RS. Management of ipsilateral supracondylar femur fractures following total knee arthroplasty. *J Arthroplasty.* 1994; 9:521–526.

16. Rand JA, Franco MG. Revision considerations for fractures about the knee. In: *Controversies of Total Knee Arthroplasty.* Raven Press; 1991:234–247.

17. Stulberg SD, et al. Case challenges in hip and knee surgery. Knee challenges: what would you do? *Orthopedics.* 1995; 18:941–947.

18. ZumBrunnen C, Brindley H. Nonunion of long bones: analysis of 144 cases. *JAMA.* 1967; 203:637.

19. Cameron HU. Double stress fracture of the tibia in the presence of arthritis of the knee. *Can J Surg.* 1993; 36:307–310.

20. Kress KJ, Scuderi GI, Windsor RE, Insall JN. Treatment of nonunions about the knee utilizing custom total knee arthroplasty with press-fit intramedullary stems. *J Arthroplasty.* 1993; 8:49–55.

21. Wilkes RA, Thomas WG, Ruddle A. Fracture and nonunion of the proximal tibia below an osteoarthritic knee: treatment by long stemmed total knee replacement. *J Trauma.* 1994; 36:356–357.

22. Schatzker J, McBroom R, Bruce D. The tibial plateau fracture: the Toronto experience 1968–1975. *Clin Orthop.* 1979; 138:94.

23. Whiteside LA. Cementless revision total knee arthroplasty. *Clin Orthop.* 1993; 286:160–167.

24. Brien EW, Terek RM, Healey JH, Lane JM. Allograft reconstruction after proximal tibial resection for bone tumours. *Clin Orthop.* 1994; 303:116–127.

25. Dennis DA. Structural allografting in revision total knee arthroplasty. *Orthopedics.* 1994; 17:849–851.

26. Mnaymneh W, Emerson RH, Borja F, Head WC, Malinin TI. Massive allografts in salvage revisions of failed total knee arthroplasties. *Clin Orthop.* 1990; 260:144–153.

27. Tsahakis PJ, Beaver WB, Brick GW. Technique and results of allograft reconstruction in revision total knee arthroplasty. *Clin Orthop.* 1994; 303:86–94.

28. Wilde AH, Schickendantz MS, Stulberg BN, Go RT. The incorporation of tibial allografts in total knee arthroplasty. *J Bone Joint Surg Br.* 1992; 74:815–824.

Index

Note: Large page ranges indicate main discussions. Page numbers followed by f indicate figures, t, tables.

A

Age considerations
  and cemented vs. cementless techniques, 99–100
  in flexion contracture casting, 63
  in tendon rupture, 154
  in total knee arthroplasty (TKA), 42
Alignment. *See* Anatomic alignment
Allografts
  for distal femur, 170–173
  invagination of, 181f, 186
  for patellar tendons, 164–167
    illustrated, 165f, 166f, 167f
  structural, 108t, 186
  See also Bone grafting
Ambulation with flexion contracture, 57–59, 66
AMK prosthesis (DePuy), 171t
Amputation, 145
Anatomic alignment
  criteria for ideal, 25
  patellofemoral, 27
  prosthetic (general), 1, 7–13
  restoration of normal, 86–88
  in sagittal and coronal planes, 1
  schools of thought on, 8
Anatomic axis
  illustrated, 9f
  measurement of, 86–87
Anderson Orthopaedic Research Institute (AORI) bone defect classification system, 117–127
  criteria of, 117–118
  definition of deficit types, 119–120
  femoral defects in, 120–127
  tibial defects in, 127–131
  "true lateral" radiographs for, 118–119
  See also Bone deficits/defects
Anesthesia, serial casting under, 62–63
Anterior cruciate ligament (ACL)
  detachment of, 63–64, 65f
  division of, 27
Anterior midline approach, 27
Anterior superior iliac spine, 18
Antibiotics
  as cement additives, 74
  for infected prosthetic joints, 150–152
AORI system. *See* Anderson Orthopaedic Research Institute (AORI) bone defect classification system
Arthrofibrosis, 147t
Arthrotomy
  medial parapatellar, 27, 39, 43, 159
  subvastus approach, 90, 159
Attenuation studies, 52

Augmentation
  blocks and wedges for bone,
    134, 138, 150–151
  for fractures. *See*
    Fractures
  modular, 37, 111
  in patellar tendon repair,
    163–164
  of quadriceps tendon,
    154–155
  radiographic visibility of,
    124–125, 131
  See also Bone
    deficits/defects; Bone
    grafting
Autografts, 81–82, 83f, 84f,
  95–96
Avulsion of tibial tubercle, 27,
  39, 158–159

B
Balancing of knee joints
  alignment concepts in, 7–13,
    25, 86–88
  with flexion contracture. *See*
    Flexion contracture
  and posterior cruciate
    ligament, 88
  soft tissue's role in, 28–31
  See also Extension gap;
    Flexion gap
Barium-infused cements, 70
Biceps femoris release, 48
Biomet prosthesis, 171t
Bleeding, 145, 147t
Blocks. *See under*
    Instrumentation/
    appliances
Blood vessels/circulation
  compromised vascular
    supply, 160
  inferomedial geniculate
    artery, 30f
  injury to, 67–68

Bone augmentation. *See*
    Augmentation; Bone
    grafting
Bone chips/slurry, 81–82, 83f,
    84f, 95–96, 172
Bone cuts. *See*
    Cutting/resection, bone
Bone deficits/defects, 116–
    132
  augmentation/grafting for.
    See Bone grafting
  classification of
    AORI system of. *See*
      Anderson Orthopaedic
      Research Institute
      (AORI) bone defect
      classification system
    defect types in, 119–132,
      122t
    history of, 116–117
    learning curve for, 132
    prerequisites for, 117–118
    radiography for, 118–119.
      *See also under specific
      defects*
  femoral
    F1 defects, 120–121, 122t,
      132
    F2 defects, 121–125, 122t,
      132
    F3 defects, 122t, 125–127,
      126t, 132
  patellar, 120
  in reimplantation, 151–152
  in revision TKA. *See*
    Revision total knee
    arthroplasty
  simple approach to, 108t
  tibial, 26f
    T1 defects, 122t, 127, 128f,
      132
    T2 defects, 122t, 127–130,
      129f, 132
    T3 defects, 122t, 130–132

Bone grafting
  autografts, 81–82, 83f, 84f,
      95–96
  followup studies on, 82
  for fractures. *See* Fractures
  intercalary grafts, 172
  preoperative anticipation of,
      27
  radiographic visibility of,
      124–125, 131
  in revision TKA. *See*
      Revision total knee
      arthroplasty
  See also Allografts; Bone
      chips/slurry; Bone
      deficits/defects
Bone loss
  augmentation for. *See*
      Augmentation; Bone
      deficits/defects; Bone
      grafting
  bone death at cement
      interface, 73
  causes of, 179
  from component removal,
      177, 179
  illustrated, 26f
  and revision TKA. *See*
      Revision total knee
      arthroplasty
  See also specific bones
Bone penetration of cement,
      72–73
Bones/bone tissue
  anterior superior iliac spine,
      18
  cortical and cancellous, 81
  death at interface area, 73
  labelling of, 82–83
  See also Femur; Patella;
      Tibia
Braces/bracing, 155–156, 161,
      167, 187
Bunnell suture weave, 161

C
Cancellous bone screws, 85,
      125, 130
Capsule, posterior, 63–65, 64f
Casting
  after tendon repair, 156, 161
  for periprosthetic tibial
      fracture, 176
  postoperative, 66
  serial preoperative under
      anesthesia, 62–63
Cementless total knee
      arthroplasty, 80–100
  alignment and kinetics in,
      86–88
  versus cemented, 77, 80, 96
  component design for,
      80–85
  history of, 7, 80
  outcomes of, 96–98
  PCL retention or
      substitution in, 88–89
  "porocoat" LCS, 54
  radiography of, 98–99
  surgical techniques for,
      90–96
  survivorship analysis of,
      96–97
Cements/cementing, 70–77
  additives to, 70, 74, 150
  barium-infused, 70
  of bone fragments, 173
  versus cementless insertion,
      77, 80, 96
  centrifugation of, 71–72, 74
  exothermic reaction of,
      71–72, 150–151
  history of, 70
  of intramedullary rods, 173
  manufacturers of, 72
  monomers and polymers,
      70–71
  and patient age, 99–100
  penetration of, 72–73

polymerization process in,
71–73
polymethylmethacrylate. *See*
Polymethylmethacrylate
(PMMA)
in revision TKA, 120, 122t,
125–127, 130, 186
techniques for, 74–77
temperature/viscosity studies
on, 71–72
See also specific components
Centrifugation of cement,
71–72, 74
Cerclage wires/sutures, 161,
166
Charnley, John, 70–71
Circulation. *See* Blood
vessels/circulation
Cobalt chrome, 81
Codivilla quadriceps tendon
lengthening, 155–156
Collateral ligaments
avoidance of resection,
63–65
medial. *See* Medial collateral
ligament (MCL)
in revision TKA, 111, 113,
115
Complications. *See under
specific procedures*
Components
alignment and kinetics in, 1,
7–11, 12f, 25, 86–88
cementless. *See* Cementless
total knee arthroplasty
constrained condylar. *See*
Constrained condylar
prostheses
design of
biologic considerations in,
80–82
geometry in, 82–85
patellar component, 85
downsizing of, 37, 38f, 172

femoral. *See* Femoral
component
infection around. *See*
Infection
intercondylar distances of
specific, 171t
loosening of, 33, 52, 73,
75, 77, 127–131, 146t,
177
migration/subsidence of,
121, 124–131, 182f
patellar tendon impingement
by, 160
porous-coated, 80–82, 83f
removal of, 171–172, 177,
179, 184. *See also*
Revision TKA
selection of, 42–43
stemmed for revision,
124–125, 128, 130–131,
151–152, 178, 182
tibial. *See* Tibial component
trial components, 107–108
See also Knee
systems/designs; *specific
components*
Condylar pegs, 75–76
porous-coated, 80–82, 83f
See also Revision TKA
Condyles
defects in. *See* Bone
deficits/defects
least-diseased, 86
osteophyte removal from,
30f, 34f, 63, 64f, 91,
95
varus/valgus effects on, 8,
10–13
Constrained condylar
prostheses, 133–147
avoidance of, 110
choice of, 182, 184
and genu valgum, 26
indications for, 26, 49, 51

as standard for fractures,
172
studies on, 42
Continuous passive motion
(CPM) machine, 49
Contractures
in flexion. *See* Flexion
contracture
postoperative, 49
with valgus deformity, 41–54
with varus deformity, 25–39
See also Releases, soft
tissue
Coonse-Adams release, 159
Coronal plane
prosthetic alignment in, 1
tibial cuts in, 14
Cruciate limitation effect, 42
Cruciate-retaining (CR)
prostheses, 33, 36, 42,
67, 76
Cuff formation, 39, 159
Curettes, 63, 184
Cutting/resection, bone
block guides for, 33–34
for cementless implants,
86–88
"clean up cuts," 184
effects on gap size, 37, 38f
equal to prosthetic
replacement, 87
instruments for. *See* under
Instrumentation/
appliances
measured, 14, 63, 91–92
of osteophytes. *See*
Osteophytes
over/under resection, 1, 2f,
36, 51
power tools for, 15–18
sharp dissection, 28–31
studies on, 88
thermal injury from, 91
See also specific bones

D
Dacron tape, 156
"Dead bone sandwich," 185
Debridement, 63, 184
Defects, bone. *See* Bone
deficits/defects
Degrees of freedom, 133
Designs. *See* Knee
systems/designs
Discharge goals after TKA,
50
Disease processes and flexion
contracture, 58, 62, 63
See also specific diseases
Dorr's classification of bone
defects, 116
Double patella, 167f
Drills, 92
Drugs
antibiotics. *See* Antibiotics
for labelling bone, 82–83
See also specific drugs
Duracon prosthesis
(Howmedica), 171t

E
Electrocautery, 17
Epicondylar axis
external rotation of, 111
femoral, 4, 10f, 11f
of femoral component, 9f,
11f
as reference point, 33f, 37,
43–44, 54
for rotational positioning, 4,
8–13
Epicondyles
axes of, 4, 9f, 10f, 11f, 111
correlation between, 12
deficits/defects in. *See* Bone
deficits/defects
definition and identification
of, 33f, 37, 43–45
exact center of, 20–21

Exposure, surgical, 27–33
quadriceps snip for, 39, 151, 159
for tibial fracture revision, 179–180, 182
Extension gap
and component positioning, 11, 12f
equal to flexion gap, 22, 35
with flexion contracture, 59–61, 60f
and posterior cruciate ligament, 88
in revision TKA, 106t, 112–113, 114f
significance of, 1–3, 4
spacers for, 37, 150–151
surgical expansion techniques, 63–66
symmetry/asymmetry of, 46
Extension of knee
casting for, 62–63
extension lag in, 155–156
with flexion contracture. See Flexion contracture
full active/full passive, 66–67
intraoperative, 185
stability/instability in, 51, 114f
trial reduction on O.R. table, 95, 113f, 185
External frames, 16f
External rotation
of femoral component, 4, 35, 37, 39, 43, 51–52, 86, 106t, 110–111
reference points for, 8
in revision TKA, 106t, 110–111

F
Femoral component
alignment of, 19–20, 45
cement versus cementless, 72–73

cementing of. See under Cements/cementing
design of, 80–82
downsized, 37, 38f, 172
epicondylar axis of, 4, 9f, 11f, 111
external rotation of, 4, 35, 37, 39, 43, 51–52, 86, 106t, 110–111
internal rotation of, 13–14, 106t, 111
lateralization of, 39
loosening of, 33, 52, 73
measuring for, 3–4, 5f
migration and subsidence of, 121, 124–127
polyethylene surface of, 81
sizing of
for primary TKA, 12f
for revision TKA, 106t, 108, 109f
valgus angle of, 4–13
See also Components; specific procedures
Femoral defects. See under Bone deficits/defects
Femoral jigs
intramedullary versus extramedullary, 19–20
standard for, 23
Femoral notching, 11, 34
Femoral shaft axis, 9f
Femur
bone loss on. See Bone deficits/defects; Bone loss
cutting/resection of, 13f, 18–21, 44–45, 66, 86–87
entry hole position in, 20f
fracture of, 140f, 143, 145, 146t
revision for, 169–173
modular augments for, 37, 111

over/under-resection of, 1, 2f,
    51
sizing of, 33
Femur periprosthetic fracture
        revision, 169–173
    challenges in, 169, 171
    hardware removal in,
        171–172
    internal fixation techniques
        for, 170–173
    intramedullary rods for, 170,
        172
    outcomes for, 173
Fibula
    head for referencing, 17
    in revision TKA, 130
Fixation
    bone screws for, 85, 125,
        130, 166
    forces on internal, 170–173
    plates and screws for, 170,
        172–173, 185
    rods for. *See* Intramedullary
        rods
    with suture, 161
Flexion contracture, 57–68
    complications of, 67
    and diseases, 57–58, 62–63
    illustrated, 58f, 61f
    outcomes for, 67–68
    overview of, 57–59
    PCL resection for, 95
    postoperative management
        of, 66–67
    preoperative evaluation of,
        59–63
    radiography of, 59, 61–62
    recurrence of, 66
    residual, 67–68
    surgical techniques for, 34,
        63–66
Flexion gap
    and component positioning,
        8, 12f

equal to extension gap, 22,
        35
    with flexion contracture,
        59–61, 60f
    and posterior cruciate
        ligament, 88
    in revision TKA, 106t, 110,
        114f
    significance of, 3, 4
    spacers for, 37, 150–151
    symmetry/asymmetry of, 1,
        5, 36–37, 46, 51
Flexion of knee
    in revision TKA, 106t,
        108–112, 114f
    stability in. *See*
        Stability/instability
    See also Flexion contracture
Fractures
    differentiation of, 175,
        184–185
    intercondylar, 173
    nonunions, malunions, and
        delayed unions of, 178,
        186–187
    patellar, 145, 146t
    radiography of, 180f
    stress fractures versus
        trauma, 175
    supracondylar, 11, 140f, 143,
        145, 146t
        revision for, 169–173
    tibial, 145, 146t
        revision for, 175–188

G
Gap size. *See* Extension gap;
        Flexion gap
Gastrocnemius muscle
    exposure of, 46
    release of, 34, 48, 63, 65f,
        66
Genesis prosthesis (Richards),
        171t

Geniculate artery, 30f
Genu valgum, 26, 45, 53
Genu varum, 26f
Gracilis tendon, 163
GUEPAR hinge, 70, 110, 126–127
Guides
    for cutting/resecting, 15–18, 16f, 22f, 33f, 34, 91
    illustrated, 167f
    intramedullary, 19–21

H
Hemarthroses, 145
Hemostasis, 171
    bleeding complications, 145, 147t
    electrocautery for, 17
Hinged knee systems, 54, 70, 110, 126–127, 133–137, 140–142
    See also specific systems
Hohmann retractors, 28–30, 31f
HSS (Hospital for Special Surgery) knee score, 97, 141–143
Humidity in O.R., 71–72

I
Iatrogenic issues, 160, 176
Iliotibial band, 45–46, 48f
Iliotibial tract "piecrust" release, 48, 159
Implants. *See* Components; Knee systems/designs; Prostheses, knee
Incisions
    anterior midline approach, 27
    complications with, 147t
    for femur fractures, 171
    lateral approach, 54
    length of, 39

medial parapatellar approach, 27, 39, 43, 159
    in revision TKA, 184
    subvastus approach, 90, 159
Infection
    antibiotics for, 150–152
    component removal with, 76, 150
    and flexion contracture, 57
    in revision failures, 145–147
    staged reimplantation for, 150–152
Inferomedial geniculate artery, 30f
Inflammation in flexion contracture, 57
Insall-Burstein prosthesis (Zimmer), 171t
Insall, John, 104, 116–117, 152, 158–159
Insall's classification of bone defects, 116–117
Instability. *See* Stability/instability
Instrumentation/appliances
    for clamping
        bone clamp, 173
        tenaculum, 39
    for cutting/resecting
        drills, 92
        guides, blocks, and slots, 15–20, 16f, 22f, 33f, 34, 91
        osteotomes, 28–31, 34, 63
        periosteal elevators, 28–31, 63
        reamers, 6, 21, 95–96, 105, 165–166, 185
        sawblades. *See* Sawblades
    for debridement
        currettes, 63, 184
    for femoral preparation, 18–20

for fixation
  bicortical screws, 166
  cancellous bone screws,
    85, 125, 130
  pins, 163
  plate and screw devices,
    170, 172–173, 185
  rods. *See* Intramedullary
    rods
  wires, 171t
history of, 7, 15–16
jigs, 19–20, 23
power tools. *See* Power tools
for retracting
  Hohmann retractors,
    28–30, 31f
  laminar spreaders, 31, 32f,
    43, 46, 54
tensors, 21–22, 54
for tibial preparation, 17–18
See also Components; Knee
    systems/designs;
    Prostheses, knee
Intercalary grafts, 172
Intermedics prosthesis, 171t
Internal rotation
  avoidance of, 4, 35, 37, 39
  of femoral component,
    13–14, 106t, 111
  and patellar tracking, 13–14
  in revision TKA, 106t, 111,
    172
  and sagittal plane, 170
Intramedullary canal
  as reference point, 11
  rod centering in, 86, 151
  size/diameter of, 19, 105
Intramedullary rods
  antibiotic-impregnated, 151
  cementing of, 86, 173
  centering of, 86, 151
  for femur fracture, 170–173
  placement of, 19
  press-fitting of, 181f, 185

for revision TKA, 106–107
size of, 12
Irrigation for cooling, 91,
    150–151

J
Jigs, 19–20, 23
Joint lines
  definition and identification
    of, 112–113
  in revision TKA, 122t,
    123–124

K
Kelikian technique of patellar
    tendon repair, 162–163
Kinematic rotating hinge
  characteristics of, 54, 110,
    126–127, 134
  illustrated, 136f, 140f
  outcomes with, 141–142
Kinematics, knee, 86–90
Kirschner wires, 171t
Knee immobilizers, 49
Knee joints, biological
  degrees of freedom in, 133
  manipulation of, 66–67
  normal alignment of, 41, 54,
    86–88
  physical examination of, 26
  varus versus valgus, 18–21
    and joint rotation, 10f,
    11f
Knee Society Scores, 67–68
Knee systems/designs,
    133–147
  AMK prosthesis (DePuy),
    171t
  Biomet prosthesis, 171t
  cementless. *See* Cementless
    total knee arthroplasty
  constrained condylar. *See*
    Constrained condylar
    prostheses

cruciate-retaining (CR), 33,
  36, 42, 67, 76
customized, 134
Genesis prosthesis
  (Richards), 171t
GUEPAR hinge, 70, 110,
  126–127
intercondylar distances of
  specific, 171t
kinematic. *See* Kinematic
  rotating hinge
low-contact stress (LCS)
  mobile-bearing, 54
MacIntosh interpositional,
  70
Miller-Galante prosthesis
  (Zimmer), 171t
Natural Knee, 85f, 97
Noiles knee prosthesis, 134,
  137f
PCL substituting, 88
"porocoat" LCS, 54
posterior-stabilized, 76, 142,
  152, 164
PROSTALAC, 151
Total Condylar III, 66, 134,
  135f, 142–143
Tricon-M, 96
variations in, 14
See also Prostheses, knee

L

Laminar spreaders, 31, 32f, 43,
  46, 54
Landmarks. *See* Reference
  points/landmarks
Lateral approach incision, 54
Lateral releases. *See under*
  Valgus deformity
Lateral retinacular release, 52,
  90, 154, 159
Lateralization of components,
  35, 39
Leg length, 172

Ligaments
  balancing of. *See* Balancing
    of knee joints
  releases of
    sequential, 1, 5, 47t, 63–65
    types of, 3, 52
    for valgus deformity. *See*
      Valgus deformity
    for varus deformity. *See*
      Varus deformity
    See also Extension gap;
      Flexion gap; Releases;
      specific ligaments
Limb length, 172
Loosening of components. *See*
  specific components
Low-contact stress (LCS)
  mobile-bearing
  prostheses, 54

M

MacIntosh interpositional, 70
Manipulation of knee joint,
  66–67
Manufacturers
  of cements, 72
  of knee systems, 134–136,
    171t
  See also specific prostheses
Mechanical axis
  forces on internal fixation,
    170
  illustration of, 9f
  measurement of, 86–87
  restoration of, 179
  schools of thought on, 8
Medial collateral ligament
  (MCL)
  attenuation studies on, 52
  contractures of, 25–28
  defective in revision TKA,
    113, 115
  illustrated, 28f, 30f
  inadvertant division of, 37

protection for, 45
release of, 28–31
superficial, 44f
varus deformity elongation
    of, 25–27
See also Releases
Medial epicondylar ridge, 44f
Medial parapatellar approach,
    27, 39, 43, 159
Medial releases. *See under*
    Varus deformity
Medialization of patella, 39,
    89–90, 92–94
Medullary canal. *See*
    Intramedullary canal
Medullary stems. *See* Pegs and
    stems
Meniscus, lateral, 27
Mersilene tape, 173
Metaphyseal region, 119–120
    deformity in, 179. *See also*
        Valgus deformity; Varus
        deformity
    fractures in. *See* Fractures
    illustrated, 118f
Methylmethacrylate. *See*
    Polymethylmethacrylate
    (PMMA)
Migration/subsidence of
    components, 121,
    124–131, 182f
Miller-Galante prosthesis
    (Zimmer), 171t
Modulus differential, 74
Monomers and polymers,
    70–71
Muscles. *See specific muscles*

N
Natural Knee, 85f, 97
Neurologic deficits/
    complications
    peroneal nerve palsy. *See*
        Peroneal nerve palsy

from vascular injury, 67–68
    vascular injury, 160
Noiles knee prosthesis
    characteristics of, 134
    illustrated, 137f
Nonunions, malunions, and
    delayed unions, 186–187

O
Osteoarthritis, 58f, 67, 81, 98f
Osteolysis
    in F2 and F3 defects, 121,
        123–131
    radiography of, 180f
    See also Bone deficits/defects
Osteonics prosthesis, 171t
Osteophytes
    flexion contracture-related,
        57–59, 58f
    lateral versus medial, 43
    osteotomes for, 34f, 63, 95
    removal of, 30f, 63, 64f, 91
    in varus deformity, 27
Osteoporosis, 76, 85
Osteotomes
    for component removal, 184
    curved, 34, 95
    for medial release, 28–31
    for osteophyte removal, 34f,
        63, 95
Osteotomy indications,
    179–180, 182

P
Patella
    defects in, 120
    double, on radiography, 167f
    eversion and dislocation of,
        27, 90–91
    fractures of, 145, 146t
    instability of, 35, 37, 39,
        51–52
    medialization of, 39, 89–90,
        92–94

radiographic tracking of, 26, 94f
as reference point, 112
resurfacing/reaming of, 6, 15, 21, 95–96, 105, 165–166, 185
in revision complications, 143, 145, 146t
thickness of, 15, 92, 98f
tracking of. *See* Patellar tracking
Patellar component
  alignment of, 14
  cementing of, 75–76
  design of, 85
  medialization of, 39, 89–90, 92–94
  positioning of, 6
  sizing of, 92
  stability of, 51–52, 87–88
  thickness of, 85f, 98f
Patellar tendon
  detachment of, 27
  disruptions of, 158–168
    allografts for, 164–167
    characteristics of, 160
    outcomes for, 168
    physical therapy/rehab for, 161–162, 164, 167
    repair techniques for, 161–168
    risk factors for, 158
    with tibial tubercle avulsion, 158–159
  forces in, 154
  impingement of, 160
  rupture of, 39, 154, 160f
Patellar tracking
  causes of maltracking, 89–90
  and femoral component alignment, 26, 51–52
  intraoperatively, 39
  and valgus deformity, 42

Patellofemoral articulation
  forces in, 8, 14–15
  stability in, 87–88
Patient selection, 81
PCL. *See* Posterior cruciate ligament (PCL)
Pegs and stems
  on cement spacers, 151
  condylar pegs, 75–76
  medullary stems, 110
  offset stems, 183f
  porous-coated, 80–82, 83f
  for revision TKA, 124–125, 128, 130–131, 151–152, 178, 182
  smooth, 82, 85
  See also specific components and procedures
Periosteal elevators
  for capsule elevation, 63
  for medial release, 28–31
Periosteum
  cuff formation of, 39, 159
  sharp dissection of, 28–31
Periprosthetic fractures. *See* Fractures; *specific bones*
Peroneal nerve palsy
  decompression outcomes for, 51
  with flexion contracture, 67
  incidence of, 147t
  from lateral releases, 50
  natural resolution of, 50, 54
Pes anserinus tendon
  detachment of, 27
  illustrated, 28f, 30f
Pes bursitis, 92
PFC prosthesis (Johnson & Johnson), 171t
Physical examinations, 26
Physical therapy/rehab. *See under specific procedures*
"Piecrust" release, 46, 48

Plate and screw devices, 170, 172–173, 185
Plumb lines, 31
Polyethylene, 14, 81, 89f, 112–113
Polymerization process, 71–73
Polymethylmethacrylate (PMMA)
  application techniques for, 74–77
  versus cementless insertion, 77
  development of, 70, 73–74
  history of, 7
  polymerization process, 71–73
  See also Cements/cementing
Popliteus tendon preservation, 48
"Porocoat" LCS components, 54
Porous coating (PC), 81–82, 83f
Posterior condylar angle, 44–45
Posterior cruciate ligament (PCL)
  in cementless techniques, 88–89
  detachment of, 63–64, 65f
  in flexion contracture, 95
  retention of, 33, 36, 91
    versus sacrifice of, 42, 88
  substitution for, 26, 88
  See also Releases
Posterior slope, 88
Posterior-stabilized knee systems/designs, 76, 142, 152, 164
Postoperative management. *See specific procedures*
Power tools
  for component removal, 184
  for cutting/resecting, 15–18
  thermal injury from, 73, 91

Preoperative planning. *See specific procedures*
Press-fitting, 181, 185
Pressurization techniques, 75
PROSTALAC (prosthesis of antibiotic-loaded acrylic cement), 151
Prostheses, knee
  alignment/angle of, 7–13
  balance of. *See* Balancing of knee joints
  constrained condylar. *See* Constrained condylar prostheses
  cruciate-retaining (CR), 33, 36, 42, 67, 76
  design history of, 7
  early failures of, 70
  Insall-Burstein prosthesis (Zimmer), 171t
  intercondylar distances of specific, 171t
  loosening of, 33, 52, 73, 75, 77, 127–131, 146t, 177
  patellar tendon impingement by, 160
  posterior-stabilized, 76, 142, 152, 164
  removal of, 171–172. *See also* Revision TKA
  stemmed for revision, 124–125, 130–131, 138, 151–152, 178
  See also Knee systems/designs; *specific components*
Prosthetic notch "plasty," 170

Q
Quadriceps muscle
  in flexion contracture, 57
  patellar expansion of, 27
  quadriceps snip, 39, 151, 159

turndown technique, 159
V-Y quadriceplasty, 39
Quadriceps snip, 39, 151, 159
Quadriceps tendon
  repair and augmentation of,
      155–156
  rupture of, 154

R
Radiography
  barium-infused cement for,
      70
  of bone defects. *See under*
      Bone deficits/defects
  double patella on, 167f
  of femur fracture, 140f
  with flexion contracture, 59,
      61–62
  misleading results of, 59,
      61–62
  of offset stem, 183f
  of osteolysis, 180f
  of patellar tendon allograft,
      167f
  of patellar tendon rupture,
      160f
  postoperative cementless,
      98f, 99f
  postoperative patellar, 26,
      94f
  preoperative, 18, 26, 93f, 98f,
      99f, 105, 179
  of revision TKA, 114f,
      179–180, 182
  subsidence on, 182f
  "true lateral" views in,
      118–119
Rand's classification of bone
      defects, 117
  See also Bone deficits/defects
Range of motion, 167, 185
Reamers/reaming, 6, 21, 95–96,
      105, 165–166, 185
Rectus muscle, 39

Recurvatum, 112–113
Reference points/landmarks
  for bone defects, 119
  epicondylar axis as, 33f, 37,
      43–44, 54
  for femoral
      alignment/rotation, 7–14,
      110–111
  for femur sizing, 5f
  fibular head as, 17
  intramedullary canal/rods as,
      11–12, 19–20
  least-diseased, 86
  patella as, 112
  of tibial plateau, 54
Rehabilitation. *See under*
      specific procedures
Reimplantation, staged,
      150–152
  outcomes of, 152
  phases of, 150
  spacer blocks for, 150–151
  See also Revision total knee
      arthroplasty
Releases, soft tissue
  Coonse-Adams release, 159
  history of, 1–3, 2t, 35
  instruments for, 28–31
  lateral, 41–54
  medial, 25–39
  over-release, 1, 2f, 36, 51, 54,
      147t
  peroneal nerve palsy from,
      50–51, 67
  "piecrust" type of, 46, 48,
      159
  See also Balancing of knee
      joints; *specific structures
      and deformities*
Revision total knee
      arthroplasty
  bone defects in. *See* Bone
      deficits/defects
  challenges in, 104–105, 115

constrained systems for, 133–147. *See also specific system names*
 complications in, 143, 145–147
 history of, 133
 illustrated, 135–141
 implant designs of, 133–138
 indications for, 138–141, 143, 145–147
 outcomes of, 141–143, 144t
with femur fracture. *See* Femur periprosthetic fracture revision
multiple, 124, 143
pegs and stems for. *See* Pegs and stems
preoperative radiography for, 179–180, 182
three-step technique for, 104–115
 extension stabilization in, 106t, 112–113, 114f
 flexion stabilization in, 106t, 108–112, 114f
 soft tissue balance in, 113, 115
 tibial platform establishment in, 105–108, 106t, 107f
with tibial fracture. *See* Tibial periprosthetic fracture revision
Rheumatoid arthritis (RA)
 and cementless components, 81
 and extension in TKA, 76
 with flexion contracture, 62, 67–68
 illustrated, 58f
 smooth central stems for, 82, 85

Robotic arms, 17
Rods. *See* Intramedullary rods
Rotation
 of epicondylar axis, 4, 8–13, 111
 excessive, 35
 external. *See* External rotation
 internal. *See* Internal rotation
 positioning for, 4
 reference points for, 7–14, 110–111
 rotational torque, 14
 stability/instability in, 186
 varus and valgus effects on, 10f, 11f
 See also specific components and procedures
Rush rods, 170

S
Sagittal plane
 forces on internal fixation, 170
 prosthetic alignment in, 1
 tibial cuts in, 14
Sawblades
 cutting blocks for, 17–18
 irrigation of, 91, 150–151
 rotating versus oscillating, 16
 thermal injury from, 73, 91
 wobbling of, 21
Screws, 85, 92, 125, 130, 166
Scuderi technique of tendon repair, 155–156
Semimembranosus muscle fluid, 29, 31
Semimembranous tendon, 31f
Semitendinosus tendon, 162–163
Sepsis, 145
Simplex cement, 75

Skin expanders, 165
Slots. *See under*
    Instrumentation
Soft tissue, 28–31
    balancing of. *See* Balancing
        of knee joints
    challenges in revision TKA,
        104–105, 115
    contraction of. *See*
        Contractures
    expanders for, 165
    over-release of, 1, 2f, 36, 51
    release of, 1–3, 2t, 35. *See
        also* Releases, soft tissue
Spacers for flexion/extension
    gaps, 37, 150–151
Stability/instability
    anteroposterior, 3
    assessment of, 36
    in flexion and extension, 51,
        113f, 114f
    of patella, 35, 37, 39
    of patellar component,
        51–52, 87–88
    rotational. *See* Rotation
    symmetric or asymmetric,
        36–37, 51
    in valgus deformity, 41
    varus-valgus, 36, 106t
    See also specific components
Staging/staged procedures,
    150–152, 177
Steinmann pins, 163
Stems. *See* Pegs and stems
Stress fractures, 175
Structural allograft, 108t, 186
Subperiosteal dissection,
    29–31
Subsidence. *See*
    Migration/subsidence of
    components
Subvastus approach, 90, 159
Sulcus, definition and
    identification of, 44–45

Supracondylar fractures. *See
    under* Fractures
Surgeons
    preferences of
        in cements/cementing, 72,
            76
        for sequence of releases,
            47t
    "surgeon's eye," 7
Surgical technique
    as central to outcome, 1
    improper, 160, 176
    See also specific procedures
Suture fixation, 161
Symmetry/asymmetry of
    flexion space, 1, 5,
    36–37, 46, 51
Synovium, 27

T
Temperature
    and cement viscosity, 71–72
    in polymerization process,
        71–72, 150–151
    thermal injury from
        sawblades, 73, 91
Tendons. *See specific tendons*
Tensors, 21–22, 54
Tetracycline labelling, 82–83
Thermal injury, 73, 91
Tibia
    bone loss on, 26f, 122–132
    cutting/resection of, 13f, 14,
        17–18, 45, 86, 88, 159
    exposure of, 27
    fractures of. *See* Tibial
        periprosthetic fracture
        revision
    normal posterior slope of,
        34, 88
    over/under-resection of, 1,
        2f
    as reference point, 54
    sizing of, 92

Tibial component
  alignment of, 13f, 14, 17–18, 52
  cementing of. *See under* Cements/cementing
  design of, 82–85
  internal rotation of, 37, 39
  lateralization of, 35
  loosening of, 75, 77, 127–131, 177
  measuring for, 5
  migration and subsidence of, 127–131, 182f
  polyethylene surface of, 14
Tibial defects. *See under* Bone deficits/defects
Tibial jigs, 23
Tibial periprosthetic fracture revision, 175–188
  allografts for, 186
  exposure for, 179–180, 182
  history of, 175–176
  incidence of, 176
  operative techniques for, 184–187
  outcomes of, 187
  physical therapy/rehab for, 187
  preoperative planning for, 179–184, 188
  staged, 177
  treatment options for, 176–178
Tibial plateau
  bone loss on, 26f, 122–132
  exposure of, 27
  with flexion contracture, 61–62
  fracture of medial, 175
  least-diseased portion of, 86
  medial subsidence on, 182f
  as reference point, 54
  slope of, 34, 88

Tibial platform rebuilding, 105–108, 107f
  See also Augmentation
Tibial trays, 76, 92
Tibial tubercle
  avulsion of, 27, 39, 158–159
  transfer of, 53
  wedge resection of, 159
Tibiofemoral alignment/angle, 8, 52
Titanium, 81, 85
TKA. *See* Total knee arthroplasty (TKA)
Tobramycin, 150
Total condylar III system
  characteristics of, 134
  high central spike on, 66
  illustrated, 135f
  outcomes with, 142–143
Total knee arthroplasty (TKA)
  age and. *See* Age considerations
  basic principles of, 1–6, 2t
  cementless. *See* Cementless total knee arthroplasty
  cements in. *See* Cements/cementing
  constraint in primary, 145
  early failures of, 70
  flexion contracture in. *See* Flexion contracture
  with fractures. *See* Fractures
  goals of, 1, 2f, 54
  infection in. *See* Infection
  neurologic complications in, 50–51, 54
  patellar tendon disruptions in. *See under* Patellar tendon
  reimplantation, staged, 150–152
  revision of. *See* Revision total knee arthroplasty
  three bone cuts in, 1, 2f

with valgus. *See* Valgus deformity
with varus. *See* Varus deformity
Tourniquets, 76, 171
Traction, skeletal
  after tendon repair, 163
  for flexion contracture, 62–63
Trial components, 107–108
Tricon-M prostheses, 96
Trochlear grooves, 82, 87
"True lateral" views, 118–119
Turnbuckle extenders, 62
Turndown technique, 159
Type 1 defects (intact metaphyseal bone), 119–121, 122t
Type 2 defects (damaged metaphyseal bone), 119, 121–125, 122t
Type 3 defects (deficient metaphyseal segment), 120, 122t, 125–127, 126f

V
V-Y quadriceplasty, 39
Vacuum environments, 71–72
Valgus angle/alignment
  of femoral component, 1, 4–13, 45
  femur cuts for, 33
  for ideal outcome, 25
Valgus deformity
  effects on femoral condyles, 8, 10–13
  femoral cuts with, 8
  implant selection in, 42–43
  lateral release for, 41–54
    bone cuts in, 43–45
    bone grafting in, 53
    complications of, 50–52
    follow-up studies on, 52–54

illustrated, 48f, 49f
    outcomes of, 52–54
    peroneal nerve palsy after, 50–51, 54, 67, 147t
    "piecrust" type of, 46, 48, 159
    postoperative management of, 49–50
    soft tissue in, 45–49
    surgeon's sequential preferences in, 47t
  and patellar tracking, 42
  pathophysiology of, 41, 54
  PCL resection for, 95
  posterior condylar angle in, 44–45
  prevalence of, 41
  sequential correction of, 1, 5, 47t
Vancomycin, 150
Varus deformity
  complications of correction, 36–39
  effects on femoral condyles, 8, 10–13
  femoral cuts with, 8
  illustrated, 26f
  ligament release indications for, 3, 95
  medial release for, 25–39
    complications of, 36–39
    intraoperative assessment of, 33–35
    outcomes of, 36–39
    preoperative planning in, 25
    techniques for, 25–35
  prevalence of, 41
Vascular supply, 30f, 67–68, 160
Vastus medialis muscle
  illustrated, 28f
  subvastus approach, 90, 159

Viscosity of cement, 71–72
Vision, 88

W

Walking/gait, 57–59, 66
Wedge resection of tibia, 159

Weight-bearing
  full, 50
  touch, 187

X

X-rays. *See* Radiography